The New Anti Inflammatory Diet for Beginners 2021

Healthy and Quick Recipes to heal your immune system

Table of content

Introduction

Inflammation is a vital part of the immune system's response to injury and infection. It is the way the body signals the immune system to heal and repair damaged tissue, as well as defend against foreign invaders, such as viruses and bacteria.

Without inflammation as a physiological response, wounds would aggravate and infections could become fatal.
An anti-inflammatory diet tops the list for controlling inflammation. Anti-inflammatory foods in vegetables, whole grains, nuts, bluefish, specific proteins, spices like ginger and turmeric, and brightly colored fruits will be substantial. I add a product to the mangosteen to fight against inflammation. Saturated fats, Tran fats, corn and soybean oil, refined carbohydrates, sugars, red meat, and dairy products promote inflammation. You can now see why, with an anti-inflammatory diet, you are also at risk of losing weight—an additional bonus.
The best thing about your diet for controlling inflammation is that it has no side effects. There is no list of side effects with most drugs. And in a few weeks, you should see an improvement.
A diet based on anti-inflammatory principles is beneficial and highly recommended. There is a study that says that this diet can protect you from disease and slow down the aging process by maintaining blood sugar and increasing metabolism.
Optimize your health with an anti-inflammatory diet.

You must integrate the anti-inflammatory principles:

High-fiber foods - Reduce inflammation by eating high-fiber foods like fruits and vegetables. You can also get it from whole grains like oats and barley.
8 servings of fruits and vegetables per day: increase your consumption of garlic, onion, leek, broccoli, cabbage, and cauliflower.
Stay away from saturated fats - Limit consumption of red meat and use herbs and spices to marinate meats to reduce toxins that form during cooking.
Avoid processed foods and refined sugar: artificial sweeteners and foods high in sodium are harmful to health and can cause inflammation throughout the body. It can also cause other illnesses like high blood pressure and increased insulin resistance.
Avoid trans fats: saturated fats are not good, just like trans fats. You should avoid these types of fats because the higher the trans fats in the body, the higher the reactive C protein, which is a marker of inflammation.
Omega-3 fatty acids: Eat foods rich in omega-3 fatty acids such as nuts, flaxseeds, and beans. You can also take omega-3 supplements, but make sure it's the best quality.
Use oils with healthy fats: organic oils like a virgin and extra virgin olive oil are good options. You can also use sunflower and canola oil. It has the best anti-inflammatory benefits.
Now that you are familiar with inflammation and what it can do for our body learn more about Instant Pot. Instant Pot will be your partner in this effort to reduce swelling.

It's a well-known fact that different foods are metabolized differently, some of which promote inflammation and others that reduce it. The anti-inflammatory diet aims to promote optimal health and healing by selecting foods that reduce inflammation. If excessive inflammation can be controlled by natural means (such as diet), this reduces dependence on anti-inflammatory drugs, which have unwanted and unhealthy side effects and do not solve the underlying problem. Anti-inflammatory medications (such as NSAIDs) are a quick fix for symptom relief. They ultimately weaken the immune system by damaging the gastrointestinal tract, which plays a significant role in the immune system's function. Blood cells and c-reactive protein. Many factors affect our body and its relationship to inflammation. So,

I think now that you have an idea of how chronic inflammation can harm your body, you are more interested in the recipes that can help you achieve a sustainable life.

Chapter 1: What is inflammation?

Inflammation is part of the body's reaction to injury or infection. It is a physiological response that alerts your immune system and needs to repair damaged cells or fight viruses and bacteria. Without inflammation to signal your immune system to work, injuries and infected sicknesses would be fatal.
Inflammation plays a role in many diseases and is associated with the immune system. We can't understand how it works, but it is evident from what you eat. Unhealthy eating adds to its causes. Get energy and limit the amount of inflammation in your body. This cookbook is not only for people who already have inflammation or autoimmune disorders but also for people who want to promote their general well-being.

The inflammation will be exacerbated in parts of the body where it is not needed. This can lead to chronic inflammation, which has been linked to stroke, heart disease, and autoimmune disorders.

There are two different types of inflammation, acute and chronic. Acute inflammation happens after an injury, such as a scratch or cut, a sprained ankle, or even a sore throat. This would cause the immune system to react only to the injured area. The inflammation would only last as long as it takes to repair the damage. This would cause the red blood vessels to dilate and increase blood flow. The white blood cells would grow in the necessary area and help the body to heal. You may see signs of acute inflammation, such as redness, swelling, pain, and the area may be warm to the touch or cause a fever.

When there is acute inflammation, the damaged tissue releases a chemical called cytokines. Cytokines act as a signal for our bodies to send white blood cells and additional nutrients to aid in healing. Prostaglandins, which are a hormone-like substance, trigger pain and fever, as well as create blood clots to help repair any damaged tissue. As the body heals, the inflammation will gradually go away until it is no longer needed.

While acute inflammation is beneficial in helping the body to repair itself, chronic inflammation can cause more harm than repair. Chronic inflammation is generally low throughout the body. A small increase often sees it in markers of the immune system in blood or tissue samples.

Chronic inflammation can be caused by anything your body thinks is a threat, whether it is or not. This inflammation will always trigger the response of white blood cells, but since there is nothing that requires your attention to heal, they sometimes begin to attack healthy cells, tissues, and organs. While researchers are still trying to understand how chronic inflammation works, it is known to increase the likelihood of developing many diseases.

Cases of acute inflammation are often easily treated with over-the-counter medications. NSAIDs and commonly used pain relievers like naproxen, ibuprofen, and aspirin are generally considered to be safe and effective for short-term inflammation. These drugs work by blocking the enzyme cyclooxygenase, which produces prostaglandins; This reduces the pain and makes it more bearable. If over-the-counter medications don't relieve the discomfort, there are prescription medications that can work just as well, such as cortisone and steroids like prednisone, which are known to reduce inflammation. Unfortunately, there are still no drugs specifically to treat chronic inflammation.

Although there are many options for treating inflammation in the short term, all drugs have side effects and may not be safe to use in the long run.

NSAIDs can increase the risk of stroke or heart attack, as well as gastric and intestinal side effects, such as ulcers and bleeding when used frequently for months or years. Cortisone can lead to weight gain, osteoporosis, diabetes, and muscle weakness. Prednisone is prescribed to treat a wide range of symptoms and illnesses, but it can also suppress the immune system and lead to an increased risk of infection. With long-term use, it can also increase the risk of osteoporosis, thinning of the skin, fluid retention, and weight gain caused by increased hunger.

Medication can work quickly and help reduce pain for a few hours, but it comes with many risks and should be taken daily, mostly several times a day, for continued relief. When the inflammation becomes chronic and affects your daily life, it's time to start looking for a safer, long-term solution to the swelling. It can be as simple as changing what and when you eat.

Processed foods

Any processed food, even partially, falls into this category. An excellent example of a partially processed food would be a dinner that comes in a box where you cook the pasta, then add the cheese to the cooked pasta. Sandwiches, potato chips, and candy are fully processed foods. This list also includes meals in the microwave, prepared meals, processed meats, cakes, bread, cold cereals, cooked meals, and any fast food.

Transfats and saturated fats

Hydrogenated oil causes inflammation because it is full of trans fats, the chemicals that make fat solid. Trans fats not only cause inflammation on their own, but they also cause inflammation by lowering good cholesterol and increasing bad cholesterol. You will find hydrogenated oils in ready-to-use baked goods like cakes, cookies, cookies, cakes, and sweet rolls. You'll also find them in fried foods, margarine, potato chips, refrigerator batter, coffee cream, and shortening. Saturated fats in the diet can also increase or cause inflammation. They can also cause imbalances in cholesterol levels and heart disease.

Alternative or artificial sweeteners

They are often used by people trying to reduce their dependence on real sugar because sugar is known to cause inflammation. But false and alternative sweeteners also have the same effects on the body as real sugar, so they are no better for your body than real sugar. These sweeteners can cause muscle pain, vomiting, fatigue, headache, abdominal pain, joint pain, nausea, mood swings, rashes, and insomnia. The only exception to this is saccharin, as it does not seem to have the same adverse effects on the body as other artificial or alternative sweeteners.

Carbohydrates

Not all carbohydrates will cause increased inflammation in your body, but some will. Many different foods are part of the food group known as carbohydrates. Glucose is a food compound that contains starch, sugar, and cellulose. You will find carbs in grains, fruits, vegetables, and milk, which are good carbohydrates. Bad carbohydrates are found in cakes, cookies, muffins, muffins, and bread. You can divide carbohydrates into two categories called complex and straightforward. Complex carbohydrates are grains, vegetables, and fruits that don't cause inflammation in your body.

When you start consuming a diet based on anti-inflammatory foods, you will notice that the inflammation already presents in your body will begin to decrease. This way of eating will also help prevent the formation of future inflammation. Everyone can enjoy the benefits of the anti-inflammatory diet. You will eat the right foods that your body needs to avoid the accumulation of inflammation and to relieve the inflammation that has already formed. The anti-inflammatory diet is based on the types of healthy foods your body needs to heal itself. Your diet will be based on fruits and vegetables, vegetable proteins like beans and nuts, whole grains, oily fish, and lots of herbs and spices to add flavor to your food.

Fruits and vegetables

All vegetables and fruits are packed with nutrients that will help eliminate or prevent inflammation, such as minerals, vitamins, and phytonutrients. These compounds are the antioxidants your body needs to fight oxidants in your body. Oxidants are also known as free radicals, cells that form during the metabolism process are released, and inflammation in your body as they work to destroy healthy cells. Free radicals will put you at an increased risk of developing chronic diseases. A type of antioxidant is found in chemicals that give fruits and vegetables their deep, vibrant color, like greens, the reds, and oranges found in a diet based on fruits and vegetables. Another type of antioxidant is known as anthocyanins; they also help fight free radicals in your body and are found in dark-colored foods, purple and blue.

Seafood, fish, and meat

Poultry and meat are rich in omega-6 fatty acids, which are the fats that cause inflammation. While there is no need to eliminate these foods, you will be healthier if you limit or even eliminate them. Most seafood and oily fish are rich in omega-3 fatty acids, which will reduce inflammation while preventing its development.

Whole grains

A grain must have all three parts intact to be called whole grain. In a piece of grain, the outer layer is the bran, the grain fiber. The middle layer is the starchy part, and the little seed inside is the part that contains vitamins and healthy fats. When the grains are refined, the healthy bran and seeds full of vitamins are discarded; the only remaining part is the starchy central part. This part contains the least amount of nutrients and causes the most inflammation when consumed without the other parts. Whole grains provide a certain amount of fiber that will feed the good bacteria that live in your gut and work to keep your digestive tract clean. Every day,

Vegetables

Legumes are packed with phytonutrients that act as antioxidants in your body and are rich in B vitamins, minerals, and fiber. All plants are right for you. They will help reduce inflammation in your body, decrease your appetite, and reduce your risk of developing diabetes, heart disease, and obesity.

Tea, coffee and dark chocolate

They are all made from plants rich in phytonutrients, and all contain caffeine known to reduce inflammation in the body. It is best to keep your coffee consumption to less than three cups a day. Tea is a better drink for the body and should be consumed frequently. When you eat dark chocolate, make sure it's seventy percent chocolate or more.

Oils and nuts

Seeds, nuts, and oils are effective in preventing or reducing inflammation in the body, but they are high in fat, which in itself can cause inflammation, so your intake should be limited to two to three tablespoons per day.

Herbs and spices

Many different flavors can be obtained through the use of herbs and spices. And many of these ingredients are known to be medicinal, so they prevent or help reduce inflammation.

You can quickly develop a meal plan based on anti-inflammatory foods. These foods will help reduce the inflammation in your body and prevent the formation of new inflammation.

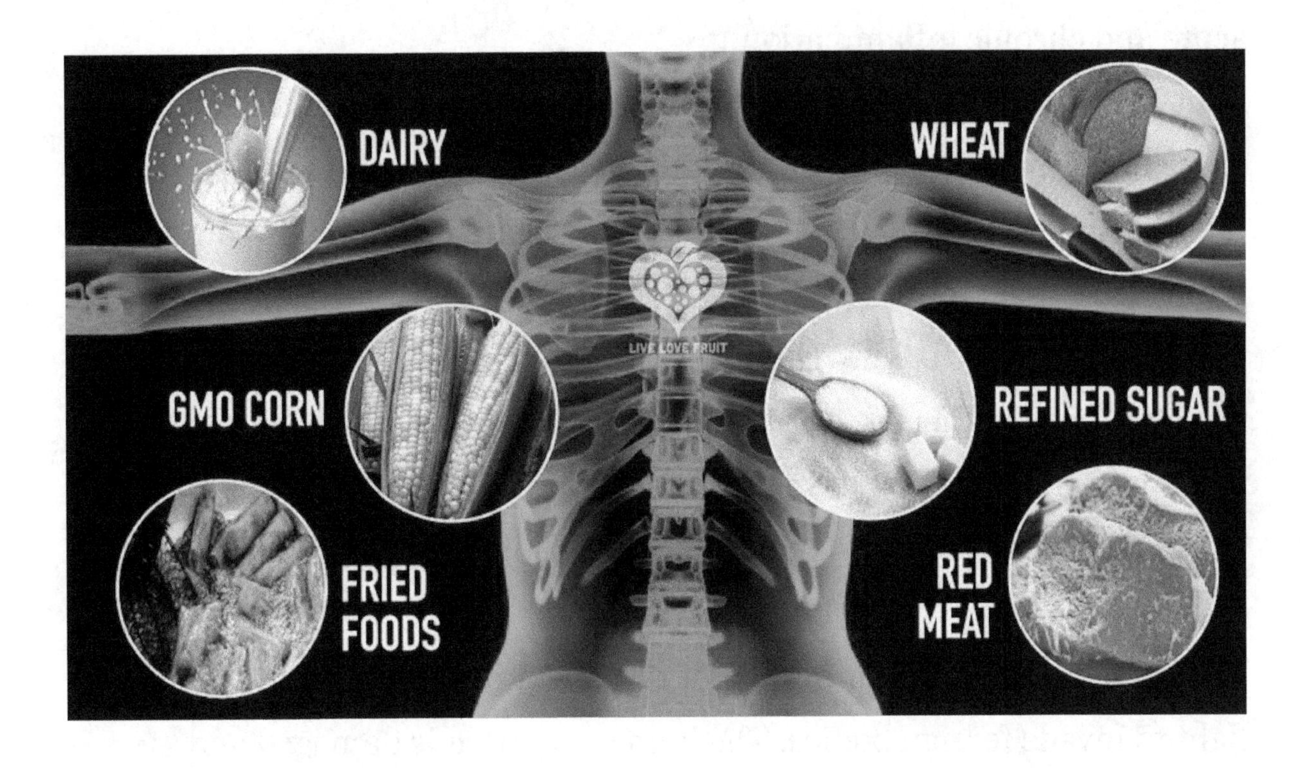

What are **Inflammation** causes?

Inflammation occurs when the body releases white blood cells to protect it from unknown substances such as contamination from a foreign entity. It is released explicitly in the injured or infected part of the body. Part of the body becomes red and inflamed because the release of chemicals affects blood flow.

There are good and bad aspects of inflammation. Yes, you read that right. Not every inflammation is terrible. There are two types of inflammation: acute and chronic inflammation.

Acute inflammation occurs when you have a sprain or sore throat. In this type of inflammation, you are assured that the body repairs itself and that the swelling will disappear when the body repairs itself. The inflammation seems to be good for the body, but there are times when the defense mechanism seems to fail. When blocked, the inflammatory response is triggered even in the absence of contamination by a foreign body. This is what happens when you have arthritis. Chronic inflammation is another story. It takes several days and stays long, leading to inflammatory diseases.

When the body has inflammation, it reacts to injuries, sending cells to fight to invade foreign bodies. The immune system is damaged and damaged. Instead of protecting the body, it causes damage and problems to the body.

Several factors cause inflammation, and one of the leading causes is related to poor lifestyle choices.

Poor nutrition: do you like to eat sweet foods? Is fast food one of your favorites? Eating unhealthy foods can trigger inflammation with fats and increased blood sugar. Poor nutrition can lead to weight gain or weight gain. It is known that having higher body fat can cause various illnesses that we don't want to have. It is essential to eat healthy to reduce our body fat. When we improve our diet, we develop it by decreasing the body's inflammatory response. This makes our bodies more efficient in managing the possible complications of our weight gain.
Aging: How aging affects inflammation remains controversial, but according to science, the progressive degenerative process is tightly integrated with inflammation. As our body ages, various cells in the body begin to die. They cannot regenerate. So when cells die, they turn to waste or foreign substances in our body that can trigger inflammation.
Lack of physical activity: Lack of physical activity can lead to obesity and overweight. There is a link between your lifestyle and your weight. Your unhealthy lifestyle can lead to changes in your physiological response to inflammatory factors. Obesity, for example, produces chronic low-grade inflammation.
Poor sleep: Getting a good night's sleep is an excellent way to start your day, but what if we lose sleep for a long time? Lack of sleep can cause physical changes in our brain and body that can lead to arthritis, periodontitis, and cancer. It can contribute to chronic diseases and mental health problems. A study shows that sleeping less than 7 to 8 hours increases inflammation. It has also been linked to chronic diseases like heart problems, diabetes, and high blood pressure.
Stress: emotional, physical, or psychological stress is not suitable for you! All of this can increase cortisol in your body. Cortisol is a hormone

produced by the adrenal glands. The higher level of cortisol can create inflammation. Studies have shown that chronic stress affects the body by altering the activity of immune cells. When you reduce stress, you live healthier. Smoking: We all know that smoking is not suitable for the body. Smoking affects and triggers an immune response to vascular damage known to be linked to high levels of inflammatory markers. The inflammatory markers are white.

Chapter 2. The science behind the anti-inflammatory diet

When your body needs to respond to an injury, it tends to mobilize an army of specialized cells to defend itself against the invading organism and toxin

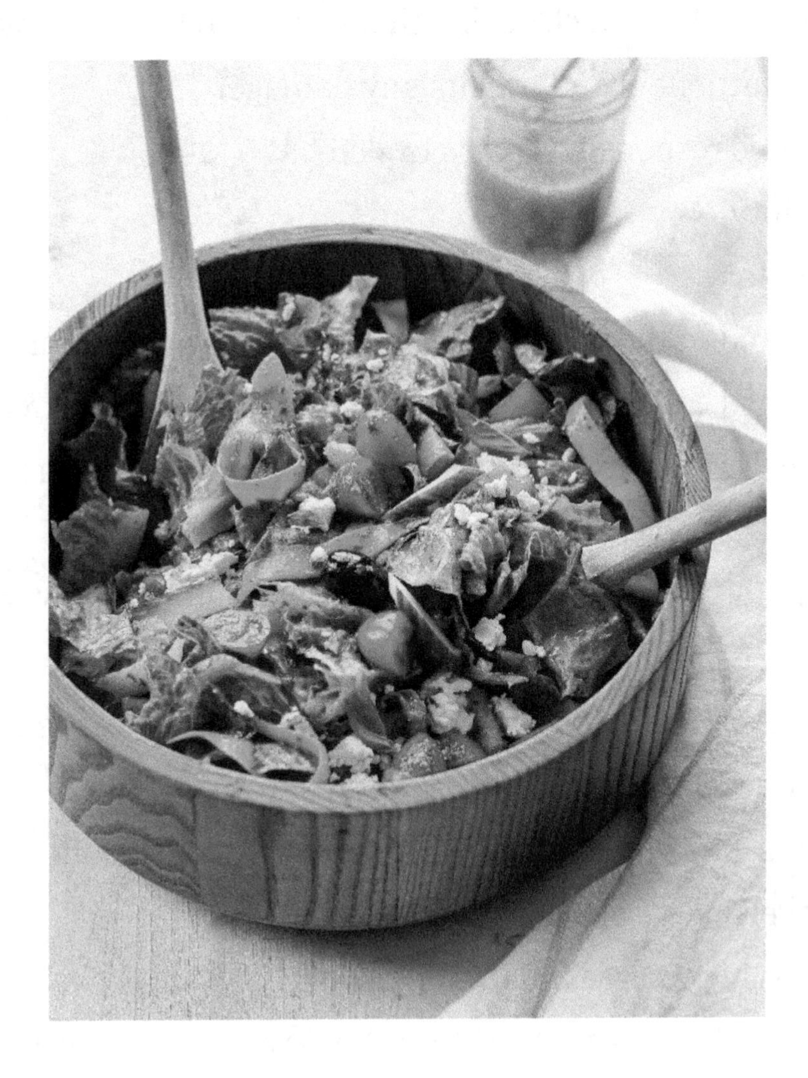

These cells prepare pathways for the combat cells to fully attack and envelop the attackers.
Once this has happened, another group of cells tends to send signals to the body and informs it that the fighting cells have completed their task and that the body can stop the production of preparatory and fighting cells.
These results are a kind of cleansing that cleans up the remains of battle cells from the battlefield and repairs any damage.
In summary, this response involves two steps:
Proinflammatory
Anti-inflammatory
Each cell involved in the professional phase builds on the work of the previous cells and contributes to strengthening the immune reaction for any future attack. During the pro period, symptoms such as redness, swelling, itching are common.
Anti-inflammatory is the opposite of proinflammatory and works to reduce the effects of inflammation.
A variety of substances used to block inflammation are made up of essential fatty acids that the body cannot make on its own.
These acids must be obtained through supplements or food.
Two essential elements are omega-3 and omega-6.
Omega-6 tends to increase inflammation, while omega-3 helps reduce it.
It should be noted that what I wrote earlier is a simplified version of the whole mechanism, and there is much more.

Several substances play a more profound role in the whole infrastructure that allows the body to control its inflammatory mechanism.

Some of the most important are:

Histamine: White blood cells near an injury tend to release a substance known as histamine. They increase the permeability of blood vessels around the wound, which signals to fight cells and other materials to regulate the immune response and detect injury. Histamine also causes redness and swelling around the affected area, creating a runny nose, rash, and itchy eyes.

Cytokines: These are proteins that are activated by proinflammatory eicosanoids to signal fighting cells to build up at the injury site. They are responsible for diverting energy from the body to catalyze the healing process. The release of these substances tends to cause fatigue and decrease appetite.

C-reactive protein: Cytokines and other pro-inflammatory eicosanoids are intimately involved in the activation of a substance known as the C-reactive protein. This particular organic compound produced by the liver responds to the messages of white blood cells. C-reactive proteins tend to bind to the injury site and act as a kind of monitoring unit that helps identify invading bodies.

Leukocytes: Several types of leukocytes (also called white blood cells) are essential to the process of neutralizing invasive substances. Neutrophils, for example, are small, agile, and can come to the crime scene first to ingest tiny germs. However, abundant materials such as macrophages are necessary to cope with a large number of microbes.

There are a few others, but the essence remains the same. When your body begins to experience an uncontrolled inflammation attack, the action of these and other similar substances tends to go haywire, which leads to extremely uncomfortable situations.

Benefits of the anti-inflammatory diet

Inflammation is the way your body protects itself from injury, illness, or infection. Your body increases the production of cytokines, immune cells, and white blood cells as a natural part of the inflammatory response. Long-term chronic inflammation often begins in your body without producing any real and noticeable symptoms. It is an inflammation that causes chronic diseases like cancer, liver disease, heart disease, and diabetes.

Inflammation is favored, or even caused, by certain factors in a person's lifestyle that is generally permanent. Some of the most damaging behaviors are regular consumption of processed foods, which can lead to insulin resistance, obesity, and inflammation. These foods will also cause diseases and conditions of the cardiovascular system.

If you want to prevent inflammation in your body or reduce the inflammation that already exists, you will need to eat more anti-inflammatory foods and fewer foods that cause inflammation. Avoid highly processed foods and base your meals on nutrient-dense foods. Your anti-inflammatory diet will give you the best combination of carbohydrates, fats, and proteins. You will want to eat certain foods and avoid others, such as:

INFLAMMATION AND FOOD

There are many causes of inflammation, including muscle tension, injuries, and illnesses. But if you have chronic inflammation, your allergies and reactions could also be caused by food.

You may have started to experience some of the above symptoms when you have eaten certain foods, as there is a direct correlation between our diet and inflammation. Hence the reason why your diet is so important.

Our bodies are designed to absorb proteins, fats, carbohydrates, vitamins, and minerals, and everything we don't need is usually eliminated from the body by the digestive system. However, some toxins cause problems because they stay in the shape when they shouldn't, triggering an immune response like inflammation to try to get rid of these toxins, which usually cause some type of damage to the body.

Toxins are more prevalent than you imagine; There are more than 100 toxins present in the body at any time. These toxins range from chemicals commonly found in various pesticides sprayed on food, food colors, specific metals that are not supposed to be in the body, and the most common toxin of all: preservatives. Preservatives are used in many food products, including some whole grain and soy products that you wouldn't normally associate with toxins or chemicals. These preservatives are used to provide a longer shelf life, whether natural (i.e., Salt) or synthetic.

Chemical preservatives are the most harmful, but the

The body has a hard time getting rid of these toxins and usually succeeds in doing so. With modern processes in food and agriculture and an increase in packaged and ready-to-eat foods, our diet today includes as

many toxins. the Day when it is almost impossible for the body to eradicate them all.
Research and studies have found that a "traditional Mediterranean" diet with a high ratio of monounsaturated fat to saturated fat and polyunsaturated fat, many fruits and vegetables, legumes, and whole grains has shown "anti-inflammatory effects compared with typical foods from North America and Europe. North ". Food models,". In general, your diet is essential for feeling better inside and out.

Chapter 3: Disease prevention

Researchers are still trying to understand the specifics of inflammation and how it affects the body, but what we do know is that inflammatory foods are linked to an increased risk of long-term and difficult-to-manage diseases, such as type 2 diabetes and heart disease.

Eating anti-inflammatory foods will calm your overactive immune system. By changing the way you eat, not only will you reduce your symptoms of inflammation, but you can even reverse the progression of conditions you already have, such as the inflammatory bowel and Crohn's disease, depression, anxiety, autoimmune diseases like lupus, psoriasis and arthritis types, cardiovascular disease, metabolic disorders like diabetes, high cholesterol, asthma and even skin conditions like eczema.

Although large-scale studies are still needed, chronic inflammation has been linked to many major diseases that affect a large part of society. Heart disease, arthritis, diabetes, Alzheimer's depression, and even cancer have been linked to inflammation. In experimental studies, it has been discovered that many foods have anti-inflammatory effects. These studies have also identified many foods and drinks that can trigger an outbreak of inflammation.

By choosing the right foods to eat, you can reduce inflammation in your body, slow or even reverse current illnesses.

Not surprisingly, most of the foods that cause inflammation are foods that we have always been told are "unhealthy". We already know that overeating unhealthy food can make us gain weight, and extra weight can increase our risk of inflammation. However, even when obesity was taken into account, there was still an undeniable link between food and inflammation.

A New Way of Life, a New You

You have the power to take control of your health. The anti-inflammatory diet aims to remove toxins and chemicals from the body from the average diet. Although it won't work in an hour or two, as painkillers will, it will reduce your chronic inflammation, increase your energy, and not have all the side effects.

When you live with chronic inflammation, do you live? By fighting chronic inflammation, it supports many symptoms that can change the way you live. He may go out less often because of pain or fatigue. You see, the world is passing and you can waste time that you could have spent with friends or grandchildren. As muscles and joints stiffen due to swelling, you may be less able to move around, even at home. This often leads to weight gain, which will only exacerbate the pain and inflammation. By consuming anti-inflammatory foods, you can reduce your pain and swell in a few days. Once your swelling is gone, you can get up and move again in no time.

It may seem challenging to drop so many of your favorite foods or go on a limited diet, but the benefits outweigh the losses. By giving up the foods that cause inflammation, you can take control of your life and your health. You will find that if you are strict and eat only anti-inflammatory foods, your taste buds will change, as will your desires.

Soon you will not miss these sweet desserts, and you will find new favorites. Once you see and feel the difference as the swelling subsides, you will not look back.

Inflammation can affect you in different ways. You may not even have realized that you are not feeling your best. This can be normal, and you didn't know you could feel stronger or faster. You may have assumed it was natural due to aging or lack of sleep. You will find that once the anti-inflammatory diet has started, your fatigue will decrease, and you will be able to sleep more deeply at night.

But to have lasting health, you have to enter it without thinking of it as a diet, but as a new way of eating, a new way of life. While inflammation can be reduced by eating the right foods, it can also return quickly if you revert to your old eating habits. You must be ready for this change. If you are tired of feeling sick and sore every day, only you can change that.

There are currently no long-term medications to reduce chronic inflammation. You may be prescribed drugs to treat inflammation symptoms, but many of these drugs have side effects and can be harmful to the liver and kidneys. These side effects can be so challenging to feel that they are now prescribing additional medications to treat the side effects of the first medication. Trying to cope with it becomes a constant battle, and the cost of drugs and doctor visits only makes it more frustrating and causes additional stress.

Make the decision to change your life for the better, eat healthy anti-inflammatory foods, and, most importantly, STOP EATING INFLAMMATORY FOOD. You will see less need for these doctor visits and these medications.

Chapter 4. What Factors to consider

The triggers for chronic inflammation can be very diverse.
However, they are often linked to each other.
It is essential to know them because learning to detect them will allow us to fight or avoid them more easily. These factors will be explained below:

Eat unhealthy food:
It is the factor that most often triggers chronic inflammation or at least the one that most easily improves its development.
The proper functioning of our body depends mainly on our diet, which must be balanced and healthy.
The reverse only modifies our body.
We must not forget that we are what we eat.
If we eat well, we will feel good, and if we do it wrong, we will feel bad. It is a reality that we have to face day after day.
The right diet translates into more energy, more stimulation, and a reduced likelihood of obesity, heart disease, diabetes, and other health threats.
A diet that lacks the nutrients necessary for our well-being and rich in fats and carbohydrates reduces our life expectancy and leads to obesity and other conditions, including chronic inflammation and all of the underlying consequences of suffering.
Cleverly, it is better to opt for the first option, right? For a healthy diet?

Unfortunately, junk food, refined flours and sugars, red meat, soft drinks, and other harmful foods tempt us easily because of their pleasant taste.
It's easy to succumb to a lousy diet, but succumbing to unhealthy foods and overeating will only lead to several illnesses that we would like to avoid.
It will also cause inflammation.
As we already know, chronic inflammation is very harmful. Its presence in our body can make us seriously ill.
Many foods commonly eaten by most people cause an incorrect, inflammatory reaction.
Our body simply does not know these "foods" as nutrients and considers them a threat. He rejects them.
The reality is that these foods are poisonous to our bodies and improve inflammation.
Here is a list of foods to prevent, prevent, and fight inflammation:
Foods that cause inflammation: refined flours
Refined sugar
Red meat
Sausages
Hydrogen oils
Snacks
Dairy products (butter, margarine, excessively fatty cheeses)
Junk food
Alcohol
And, in general, processed foods.
Reducing the consumption of these foods is vital in the fight against inflammation and its prevention.

Overweight:

Obesity and inflammation are linked.

Chronic inflammation produces obesity and vice versa.

The truth is that being overweight generates inflammatory reactions in the gut, abdomen, and the body in general.

If we do nothing, the inflammatory reaction caused by obesity will stay in our bodies longer than it should, and the dreaded chronic inflammation will appear.

This factor is closely related to that explained above.

A diet based on flour, refined sugar, and other unhealthy foods, such as those with excess fat or carbohydrates, will cause obesity and chronic inflammation.

This establishes the importance of a healthy diet to avoid inflammation and its diseases.

.

Sedentary life:

This factor that triggers chronic inflammation is linked to the previous ones.

Poor nutrition and a sedentary lifestyle will lead to the development of obesity and, as a result, chronic inflammation.

When you lead a sedentary life, your body is not functioning correctly because we are not helping you get proper oxygenation. As a result, the immune system is likely to weaken and not work as well.

The weakened immune system will have to work harder to fight the harmful agents and external agents that can make our bodies sick.

This can undoubtedly lead to chronic inflammation.

To smoke:

It's no secret that smoking is harmful to health and one of the leading causes of death worldwide.

This bad habit significantly damages our lungs, promotes cancer, and the onset of inflammatory diseases like gingivitis, rhinitis, and the like. It also hurts our dental health by contributing to the weakening of the teeth.

Not to mention the lousy breath smokers face.

Some people think that the adverse effects of smoking are only those mentioned above.

But they are wrong.

Smoking also improves chronic inflammation.

When we smoke, we let our lungs be bombarded with cigarette smoke or tobacco.

Our brain detects the presence of this smoke as an invasion, and, in response, our immune system activates the inflammatory process.

If we smoke too often, the body will start the process just as often, and sooner or later, the acute inflammation will become chronic.

Pollution:

Another trigger for chronic inflammation is pollution.

Another trigger for chronic inflammation is pollution.

With pollution, something similar happens with what happens with the action of smoking.

Exposure to pollutants often activates our immune system to protect us from anything it considers invasive: smoke and bacteria that can adhere to us in the garbage. These viruses circulate in polluted air, among others.

Over time, this body's natural reaction will become chronic as it has been activated for too long or repeatedly.

Change your body and mind.

You will notice immediate changes in your body and mind when you start consuming an anti-inflammatory diet. Your skin will be lighter and smoother than ever. Your joints will be less painful when you begin to lose weight. Your cravings for sugar and fatty foods will disappear. You'll move better, sleep better, and think more clearly than ever. Many of the chronic diseases that humans suffer from are caused in part by inflammation, and many of these same chronic diseases cause inflammation. People suffering from any of these diseases would greatly benefit from following an anti-inflammatory diet.

Type 2 diabetes

- Thyroid disease
- Rheumatoid arthritis
- Psoriasis
- Osteoarthritis
- Obesity
- Metabolic syndrome
- Lupus
- Inflammatory bowel disease
- High cholesterol
- Hypertension
- Eosinophilic esophagitis
- Crohn's disease

- Colitis
- Asthma

When planning your anti-inflammatory meals, remember the following:

Eat all the rainbow colors to make sure you eat food with all the nutrients you need.

Simple, fresh ingredients are best for you because even a little processed food can change their nutritional content.
There is no such thing as "magic" food that suddenly improves your health. This is why eating the rainbow is crucial because you need many varieties of food to get its nutrients.
Whenever you use pre-prepared foods carefully, check the labels for added fats and sugars.

Some foods are more anti-inflammatory than others simply because of the nutrients they contain. Here are thirteen of the best foods to fight inflammation.
Cherries
Cherries are full of antioxidants that will help fight inflammation in your body.

Coke and dark chocolate
In addition to helping satisfy the craving for something sweet, dark chocolate is an excellent source of antioxidants that will help reduce inflammation. The anti-inflammatory benefits are found in the

antioxidants known as flavanol, which, in addition to fighting inflammation, will help keep the cells in your arteries healthy.

Turmeric

This spice is widely used in Indian dishes such as curries. It is the spice that contains curcumin, which is a potent anti-inflammatory. And when you combine the curcumin in turmeric with the piperine found in black pepper, you have a fantastic weapon that will help decrease the inflammatory markers in people with chronic inflammation.

Mushrooms

These are full of B vitamins, copper, and selenium, all anti-inflammatory while being very low in calories. Mushrooms are best eaten lightly cooked or raw for all their benefits.

Green tea

With its anti-inflammatory and antioxidant properties, green tea is one of the best and healthiest drinks you can drink.

broccoli

It is a cruciferous vegetable which, along with other cruciferous plants, will help reduce the risk of developing chronic diseases. And broccoli is rich in antioxidants that will fight inflammation in your body by lowering the cytokines responsible for inflammation.

Berries

These berries are full of minerals, vitamins, and fiber. People who eat seeds regularly have a more functional immune system.

Oily fish

Oily fish contain compounds that reduce inflammation, which can lead to kidney disease, diabetes, heart disease, and metabolic syndrome.
And fatty fish is full of omega-3 fatty acids.

Lawyers

These are one of nature's pure superfoods because they contain antioxidants and heart-healthy fats, fibers, magnesium, and potassium.

Peppers

Peppers and peppers are loaded with antioxidants and vitamin C.

Grapes

Grapes are a great source of the antioxidant resveratrol, along with other antioxidants, which help reduce inflammation and the risk of developing eye disorders, Alzheimer's, obesity, diabetes, and heart disease.

Olive oil

It is one of the healthiest fats you will consume in the anti-inflammatory diet. It is loaded with monounsaturated fats and will help reduce inflammation.

Tomatoes

These are rich in lycopene, an anti-inflammatory antioxidant, potassium, and vitamin C. If you cook your tomatoes in olive oil, you will double the benefits of lycopene.

Eating a specific type of anti-inflammatory diet is the best defense for reducing inflammation in your body. It can also help improve or lessen the effects of certain chronic diseases. A diet rich in healthy fats, whole grains, nuts, seeds, vegetables, and fruits will help improve many chronic diseases by relieving chronic inflammation.

Chapter 5. Signs of inflammation.

The main signs of inflammation are warmth, redness, pain, swelling, and loss of muscle function. These signs depend on the inflamed part of the body and its cause. Some of the prevalent symptoms of chronic inflammation are:

- Frequent infections
- Weight gain - Body pain.
- Insomnia
- Tired
- Mood disorders, such as anxiety and depression.
- Gastrointestinal issues like diarrhea, constipation, and acid reflux.

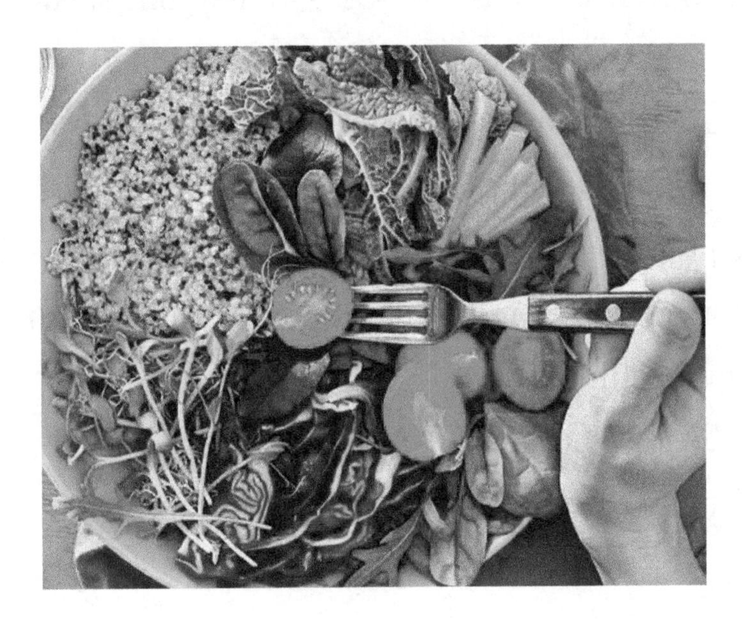

Typical signs of inflammation depend on various problems of inflammatory effects. When the body defends the mechanism that influences the skin, it causes rashes. As for rheumatoid arthritis, it affects the joints. Most of the signs and symptoms experienced include fatigue, tingling, joint pain, stiffness, and swelling.

Likewise, when an inflammatory bowel is felt, it generally influences the digestive system. Its usual signs are hemorrhagic ulcers, anemia, weight loss, bloating, body aches, diarrhea, and upset stomach. With multiple sclerosis, the condition occurs in the myelin sheath, which covers the nerve cells. Its signs include stool problems, double vision, blurred vision, fatigue, and cognitive issues.

If you experience any of the above signs and health problems, you may be suffering from inflammation. Many people associate it with joint pain, such as arthritis pain, which can be indicated by swelling and pain. The problem is related to health issues, not just swollen joints. However, not all pain is bad. For example, acute inflammation is vital when recovering from a sprain and ankle sprain.

It is easy to detect the signs and causes of chronic inflammation. Insomnia, genetic predisposition, food intake, and other individual habits can be the cause. Likewise, the inflammation resulting from an allergy can also develop in the intestine.

Here are some of the possibilities it can have;

- If you still feel tired to the point of not getting enough sleep, not getting enough sleep, or getting too much sleep.
- Do you have occasional aches and pains? It can also mean that you have arthritis.
- Do you have stomach or stomach pain? The pain can create inflammation. Intestinal inflammation can also cause cramps, bloating, and loose stools.

- Another sign of inflammation is a swollen lymph node. These nodes are located in the neck, armpits, and groin, which swell when there is a problem in your system. When you have a sore throat, the knots in your neck increase because the body's defense system has detected the condition. These lymph nodes react when the body fights infection. The nodes are reshaped as they heal. - Do you have a stuffy nose? This can be a symptom of irritation of the nasal cavities.
- Sometimes your epidermis may protrude due to internal inflammation.

BENEFITS OF FEEDING

The anti-inflammatory diet is used to reduce the amount of inflammation in the body by eliminating the foods that usually cause swelling, reducing the symptoms experienced, and improving overall health. The benefits of the anti-inflammatory diet are revealed below:

REDUCE THE RISK OF EXPERIENCING MORE ILLNESSES OR DISEASE

Reducing your inflammation will reduce your risk of suffering from one or more of the problems mentioned above, including obesity and allergies. If you are at risk for heart disease, predisposed to diabetes, have high blood pressure, or even stiff and painful joints, this diet is for you. This will help reduce inflammation, and you should feel much better over time.

LOSE OR KEEP A HEALTHY WEIGHT

Likewise, if you are trying to lose weight, you may not have considered typically inflammatory foods as the problem, as they are not always associated with weight gain. Instead, you may have tried to control your calorie intake and exercise more while struggling to lose weight. Now, this is not a fad diet, and you probably won't miss a pants size in two weeks. But that is not the purpose of this change, as there are many more benefits to gradually losing weight and changing your eating habits in the long run. The healthy foods used in this cookbook will help you lose weight and reduce inflammation.

PREVENTING FOOD ALLERGIES

As previously stated, the anti-inflammatory diet can also contribute to food allergies. Allergies can be problematic for many people and, if they are severe enough, they can be life-threatening. Reducing inflammation can help minimize the severity or regularity of the allergic reactions you experience.

EXCELLENT FOR GLUTEN FREE

For many people allergic to gluten, this book can also help. Often people do not recognize gluten as a problem until they follow this diet or a gluten-free diet. The anti-inflammatory nature of this diet can help alleviate the symptoms experienced by those who are gluten intolerant.

IMPROVE YOUR SKIN

Along with all of these benefits, diet can also significantly improve the skin.

Sometimes the inflammation can cause dry, aged skin, and you may also have noticed redness and even problems like rosacea on the surface, all of which can be caused by inflammation. This diet can help improve the appearance of your skin, which means you will feel and look younger!

INCREASE YOUR ENERGY LEVELS

Also, your energy will increase. Sometimes we can feel our energy drained due to the foods that cause inflammation. Not only do sugars deplete our power, but also processed foods. You are what you eat as the old saying goes, and sometimes eating foods that cause fatigue and tiredness can be a significant problem. These foods can also depress you. However, with the inflammation diet, you can say goodbye to lethargy and depression by eating foods that give you energy and improve your quality of life.

REDUCE SYMPTOMS

Then there is the pain and the pain that you feel. You shouldn't have to live with chronic pain, and if you don't eat the right foods, your symptoms will undoubtedly be worse than necessary. Pain shouldn't take over your life, and you can make sure it doesn't go through the foods and meals recommended in this cookbook.

BE THE HAPPIEST AND HEALTHIER VERSION OF YOURSELF

Making your own informed decisions can change your life for the better. Try this diet, and you will soon realize the potential of your body and mind, and what you have missed. Don't let your health get in the way - eat well, live well, and be well!

Chapter 6. Foods that naturally reduce inflammation:

There are many options to avoid the multitude of harmful products that contain inflammation-producing agents that can be divided into several categories when it comes to eating with an eye on anti-inflammatory foods. Engage in the following guidelines for the foods you should eat and the foods you should avoid in your memory, and you will be free from inflammation in no time.

Eat more fiber: Studies show that a high fiber diet will naturally create a lower overall level of inflammation due to all the phytonutrients that unprocessed natural foods, including fruits and vegetables, have in swords. To make sure you consume 25 grams of fiber a day, be sure to eat lots of blueberries, 3.5 grams of bananas, and 3 grams of onion, eggplant, okra, oats, and barley.

Aim for nine servings of vegetables and fruit each day - be sure to consume a 2: 1 ratio of vegetables to fruit, because too much fruit can quickly increase your total sugar intake. One serving is generally considered to be half an ac of cooked vegetables or 1 tsp of raw vegetables. Ginger and turmeric are known to fight inflammation, and both are excellent condiments.

Aim for four portions of crucifixes and alliums each week: alliums are like leeks, onions, chives, and garlic. At the same time, crucifers include many vegetables, such as Brussels sprouts, mustard, cauliflower, cabbage, and broccoli. All of these contain incredibly high antioxidants, so a few per week are enough to significantly reduce the risk of cancer linked to

inflammation when consumed regularly. Remember, four servings a week is the minimum for alliums and crucifers, the crazier one is.
Keep saturated fats to a minimum: To start actively reducing the amount of inflammation in your body, it's essential to monitor the amount of saturated fat you consume daily carefully. This means reducing it to 10 percent of the total amount of calories you consume in a day. This means that you will probably want to cut down on red meat and stick to healthy marinades made with anti-inflammatory spices instead of coconut oil.

Eat lots of omega-3 fatty acids: As discussed above, eating more omega-3 fatty acids should be at the top of the list for anyone who wants to reduce their level of inflammation. In addition to being found in fish, it is also found in high doses in nuts, flax and soy, kidneys, and white beans. A regular omega-3 supplement is also recommended. When it comes to fish, anchovies, sardines, trout, mackerel, herring, oysters, and salmon all contain the highest amounts of omega-3, and you should be consuming 3 per week. Look for healthy fats: fats have had a bad reputation over the years because, at one point, the dominant society decided to group all the fats. Healthy fats are a good source of energy for those who avoid carbohydrates in favor of a more natural energy solution. This means that many healthful fats, such as those found in coconut oil, coconut oil, and pressed canola oil, are a great way to eat healthy inflammatory elements and rinse your system at the same time. Avoid products made with corn syrup and refined sugar: studies show that simply adding a daily dose of processed foods to your diet by eating things that are dosed in large amounts of sugar or corn syrup is enough to increase their inflammation levels dramatically

Avoid trans fats: in addition to saturated fats, it is essential to avoid fats as often as possible. This means looking at product labels because trans fats are often hidden under partially hydrogenated oils. Trans fats are known to cause inflammation in the cell wall of the arteries, as well as lower levels of beneficial cholesterol, which increase that of the harmful variety.

Avoid the wrong types of oil: In general, the healthy fat-based fats listed above are a healthy option, all others should be avoided no matter what health claims they may promote. These oils are often extracted using chemicals known to increase inflammation. They are rarely disclosed on product labels because they are used in product creation and are not added after the fact. They also tend to be rich in omega-6 fatty acids, which decreases the body's balance between that and omega-3 fatty acids and increases inflammation in the process.

Avoid refined carbohydrates: while complex carbs are an excellent source of energy, refined sugars are generally simple carbohydrates, which means that they break down extremely quickly and are at the same time responsible for the feeling of low energy related to an accident. Sugar. Also, the refining process is just another word for processing, which means it takes away the little nutritional value they would otherwise have. They also tend to be high in sugar, making them a trigger for inflammation in almost every conceivable way.

Avoid excess alcohol: When consumed in excess, beer, and hard-drinking have been linked to increased inflammation if used regularly. A good rule of thumb is that men should not consume more than two glasses per day and women should limit themselves to 1 glass if they want to drink, while keeping their level of inflammation to a minimum.

Overuse of anti-inflammatory drugs can cause harmful side effects for the body. Therefore, the best option to fight inflammation is to do it through food.

Many foods have anti-inflammatory or antioxidant properties that can help us eliminate inflammation or prevent it naturally.

These foods are useful in reducing the bothersome symptoms present in acute inflammation and minimizing the likelihood of suffering from chronic inflammation or reducing the after-effects it can cause in the body.

These precious foods and their specific health benefits are explained below: - List of anti-inflammatory foods 1 - Foods rich in Omega 3:

Oily fish:

- Wild salmon
- Trout
- Sardines
- Anchovy
- Mackerel
- 2.- Seeds:
- Linseed
- Chia seeds:
- Sesame seed:
- Hemp: sunflower seeds Fruits:

- Pineapple
- lemon
- Strawberries
- Blueberries
- Papaya grapes
- Guava
- Lawyer
- Kiwis
- Dried fruits:
- Nuts
- Hazelnut
- Vegetables
- broccoli
- Tomatoes
- cauliflower
- Carrot
- Garlic
- Onions
- Salad
- Chard
- spinach
- Legume Radishes
- Soy peas
- Chickpeas
- Green beans Black beans
- Natural oils
- Olive oil linseed oil

- Avocado oil Coconut oil Spices:
- Turmeric
- Ginger
- Cinnamon
- Whole grain
- Oats
- quinoa
- Fermented foods
- Kombucha
- Kefir
- Miso
- Mushrooms
- Infusions
- Green tea
- Matcha tea
- Lean meats
- List of anti-inflammatory foods and their health benefits 1 - Foods rich in Omega 3: Oily fish:
- Wild salmon
- Trout
- Sardines
- Anchovy
- Mackerel
- herring

The variety of foods mentioned above is an essential source of omega-3 fatty acids or healthy acids.

Omega-3s in medical science is effective in fighting arthritis symptoms, reducing asthma symptoms, and preventing heart disease.
Their significant contributions to the improvement of the diseases mentioned above are because these acids are effective in reducing high cholesterol levels, and they have anti-inflammatory effects.
This nutrient is considered essential for preventing or fighting chronic inflammation.
In addition to the above, these foods provide a significant amount of protein to the body.
They are the perfect substitute for red meat, excessive consumption of which can have serious health consequences.
They are ideal for including in any meal. Breakfast, lunch, or dinner can be accompanied by many other healthy foods, such as any existing variety of vegetables or mushrooms. It is best to eat them grilled or baked.
Linseed
These are seeds that are very popular in diets and in cooking in general. These are seeds with important medicinal properties.
Flax or flax seeds are seeds of high nutritional value that we can get the most out of.
Within anti-inflammatory diets and even within weight-loss diets, its presence is essential.
Among all the edible seeds, they are among the healthiest and most favorable.
They contain high levels of fiber, healthy fatty acids such as omega 3, which are present at least 55% of its nutritional content, vitamins such as vitamin E and various minerals such as phosphorus, iron, potassium, and others.

They also contain essential contributions of vegetable proteins.
In our body, they exert a laxative effect, which keeps our stomach clean and has antioxidant and anti-inflammatory effects in general. They are also known to have promoted digestion by reducing the time of intestinal transit.
At the same time, they are highly dietary and can be included in any slimming diet.
Adding a handful of these seeds to drinks and salads is enough to take advantage of their incredible benefits.
One of the most common ways to consume them is to add them to a glass of water and drink it.
In this simple way, we prepare a refreshing and highly nutritious drink with a satiating effect, which will help us to avoid harmful temptations and fight the dreaded chronic inflammation.
- Chia seeds:
Adding a handful of these seeds to salads, smoothies, and other recipes will significantly improve our health.
Chia seeds are considered a superfood, which means that they contain many nutrients.
Their high concentration of mucilage (a type of healthy fiber) makes them ideal for promoting the proper functioning of the immune system because they help purify the body.
These substances lubricate the gastrointestinal tract, facilitating intestinal transit. Therefore, they fight constipation and cleanse us of toxins.
A small handful of them contains about 12 grams of this fiber, which is so beneficial in anti-inflammatory diets.

In addition to fiber, it contains antioxidants and various minerals such as calcium or boron. They also contain omega 3.
Its consumption allows us to comply with at least 3 of the principles of anti-inflammatory diets: higher consumption of omega 3, a greater use of soluble fiber, and consumption of anti-inflammatory foods. There is no doubt that these seeds are potent anti-inflammatory foods capable of limiting the ravages of chronic inflammation and reducing the symptoms of acute inflammation, which are bothersome.
There is no excuse for not including them in your diet. Spread them over your salads and drinks, and your health will be very grateful to you.
Hemp:
Hemp seeds are considered a macronutrient because of their high content of vitamins, minerals, and other components.
They are rich in magnesium, iron, essential fatty acids, protein, vitamin E, and fiber.
Thanks to fiber, they have laxative effects that improve the digestive system and the secretion of impurities, helping the body to cleanse itself.
Thanks to their vitamin E content, they fight against free radicals, oxidation, and inflammation.
Thanks to their fatty acid content, they also improve the symptoms of many inflammatory diseases due to their inhibitory quality of the inflammatory process.
Sunflower seeds:
These seeds are found in the center of the flower called sunflower.
They are safe to eat and very rich in nutrients.

They are effective against inflammation and are attributed to improving the symptoms of inflammatory diseases such as asthma and rheumatoid arthritis because they contain high values of vitamin E.
You can eat them with yogurt with nuts and other seeds, include them in salads or salad dressings and even smoothies.

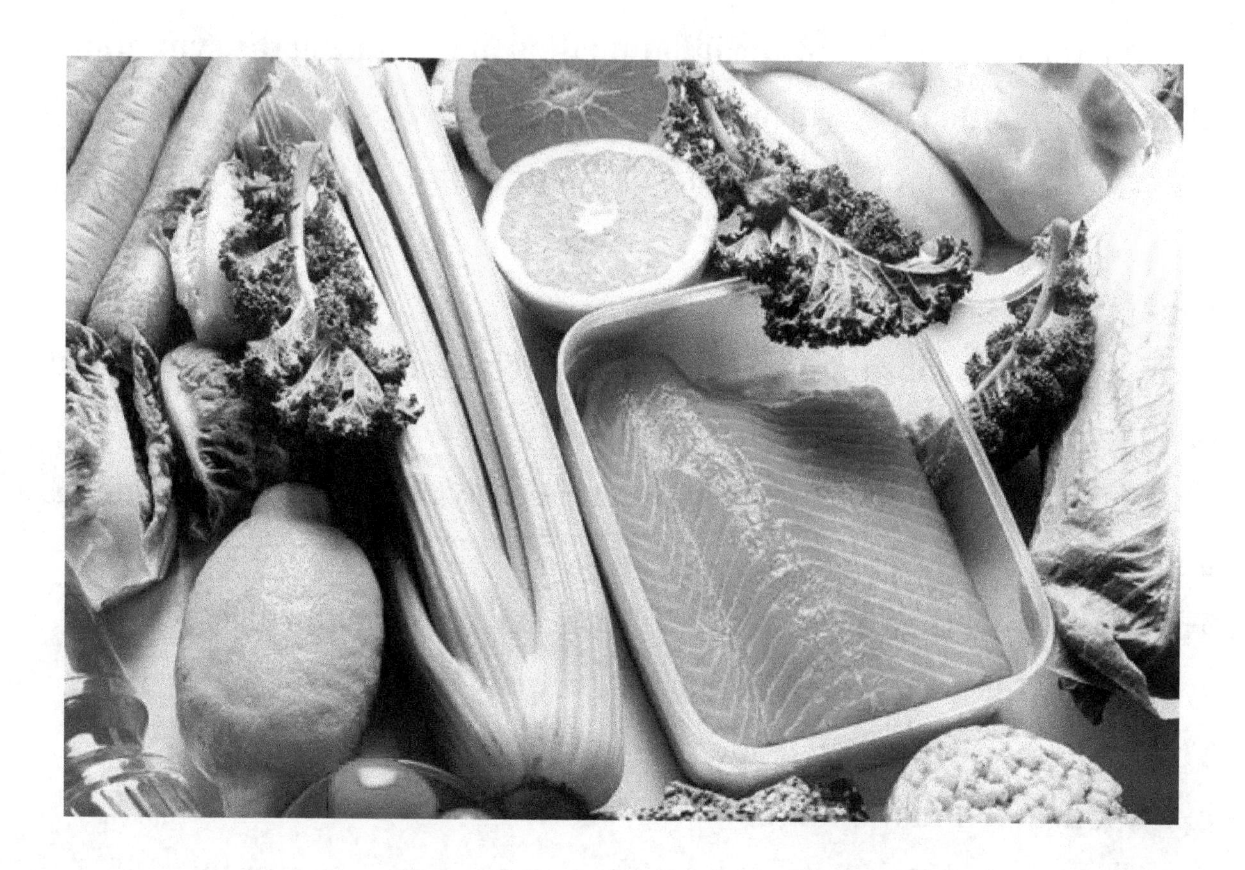

Chapter 7. Common misconceptions about the anti-inflammatory diet

There is no exact definition of an anti-inflammatory diet, and the meaning depends on who you ask. Therefore, there are many misconceptions about this diet. We will clarify some myths so that you can get rid of them and focus on what matters to improve your health.
Some of the main misconceptions and mistakes regarding the anti-inflammatory diet are:
An anti-inflammatory diet is a restrictive diet.
People who try to control their diet for one reason or another often end up with rigorous diets. They create a list of foods to avoid and end with joyless diets that can also compromise your nutritional intake. Sometimes very restrictive diets can even cause more health problems than they help.
The truth is that anti-inflammatory diets are made up of a wide variety of foods and only work to limit the amount of ingestion rather than eliminating food from your diet. This ensures that you enjoy tasty meals in the right amounts without having to overthink about restricting food.
Spicy foods cause inflammation.
This misconception comes from the Middle Ages. Many people believe that spicy foods are the cause of many health problems. The truth is that some spices can make certain medical conditions worse, but there is no scientific evidence that spices cause disease. Therefore, when planning your anti-inflammatory regimes, consider that each food substance is included rather than following such generalizations.
There is only one recipe for all anti-inflammatory diets.

This is another misconception about the ability of many people to use anti-inflammatory diets. The truth is that different people suffer from different types of inflammation caused by different agents. So what works for one person may not work the same way for another person. There are many conditions involved with inflammation, which can affect how your body reacts to certain foods. It is important to keep this in mind and experiment with various foods until you find what works for you. If you try a specific diet and find that it doesn't work for you, give up the whole problem and try other different foods to see if

Milk causes inflammation.

Many reports suggest that milk is bad for our health. Among the central claims in these reports, milk causes inflammation. However, studies have shown that milk and other dairy products have anti-inflammatory properties and can protect against chronic inflammation. Therefore, it is important to consider including milk in your anti-inflammatory regimes, as it has been shown to have substantial health benefits.

Chapter 8. What type of disease can cause inflammation?

If we make a comparison, we will see that most of the inflammation causes are related to diet, so we keep it at the top of the list. Harmful substances like refined fats, animal products, and refined carbohydrates cause long-term damage. However, it should be noted that sugars do not directly contribute to inflammation. However, processed foods with a higher concentration and fats are naturally dense with inflammatory substances that affect the intestine and increase inflammation.

The types of fat consumed by an individual also play a role here. At first, when everything was simple, people followed a balanced diet of omega-3 and omega-6 fats. However, fresh foods tend to have a high concentration of omega-6 fatty acids compared to omega-3 fatty acids; This increases the risk of inflammation by 10-20%. The body needs to have a good supply of omega-3 fatty acids because omega-6 and omega-3 both compete for the same COX enzymes needed to build large fat molecules. The COX-2 enzyme, in particular, is essential for the production of inflammatory prostaglandins. Too much omega-6 fatty acids will control this enzyme, and the body will no longer be able to use the protein in conjunction with omega-3 fatty acids to reduce inflammation. Today, fats are chemically modified, which also plays a more significant role in inflammation.

They are made to be less expensive, which results in the production of highly inflammatory products. Aging The natural process of aging also contributes to inflammation. As we age, our cells can regenerate, but most of them start to die, leaving waste products that can cause inflammation.

Obesity and inactivity Excessive inactivity can often lead to obesity, which is a significant cause of inflammation. Adipose tissue, the layer of fat just below our skin, is responsible for much more than just keeping it warm. It is a metabolically active layer that causes the body to change its chemistry and is also affected by other systems in the body.
The fat layer contains a large number of white blood cells and a higher level of fat. The number of cells is related to each other. That is, the more fat there is, the higher the number of white blood cells present. These cells often release pro-inflammatory substances, which gradually contribute to the increase in inflammatory effects. Sleep deprivation Researchers have shown that lack of sleep is linked to the formation of specific white blood cells that fight infections, such as T lymphocytes.
Depriving us of sleep will decrease the number of T cells, which will increase the number of cytokines that promote inflammation. Stress Cortisol is a hormone produced by the adrenal glands and is used to control the body's response to stress. It helps stimulate energy explosions and removes pro-inflammatory substances.
It also helps reduce stress by neutralizing the effects of pro-inflammatory eicosanoids. However, if you become too stressed, the amount of cortisol can increase to a dramatic level, which will cause your immune cells to lose sensitivity to this hormone and trigger inflammation. Sun exposure may sound a bit surprising, but excessive sun exposure can often cause inflammation. Sunburn or overexposure promotes the formation of free radicals below the surface of the skin. To let you know, free radicals are unstable molecules that tend to destroy injury-fighting cells and reduce the number of white blood cells in the body. As you may have guessed,

Smoking Exposure to various toxins, such as cigarette smoke, plays a vital role in inflammation. Whether used or first-hand, inhaled tobacco tends to weaken the body's ability to fight disease by suppressing the production of white blood cells. The madness behind inflammation So why are people going for an anti-inflammatory diet? Despite the best health care technologies and services worldwide, the United States suffers from an epidemic of chronic inflammation and other chronic inflammatory diseases.

The change in the form of a modern diet also contributes to increasing the number of incidents. When we talk about chronic inflammation, we imply various diseases like arthritis and asthma among the long term illnesses/diseases. Inflammation Science Now that you have an idea of the severity of the inflammation due to a problem, let's take a look at how inflammation works and what happens to your body during inflammation. When your body needs to respond to an injury, it tends to mobilize an army of specialized cells to defend itself against the invading organism and toxins. These cells prepare pathways for the combat cells to fully attack and envelop the attackers.

Once this has happened, another group of cells tends to send signals to the body, informing it that the fighting cells have completed their task and that the body can stop the production of combat and preparation cells. This results in a kind of cleansing that cleans up all of the remaining battle cells on the battlefield and repairs any damage. In other words, there are two stages to this response: pro-inflammatory and anti-inflammatory. Each cell involved in the professional phase builds on the work of the previous cells and contributes to strengthening the immune reaction for any future attack. During the pro period, symptoms such as redness, swelling, itching are common. Anti-inflammatory is the opposite of pro-inflammatory,

A variety of substances used to block inflammation are made up of essential fatty acids, which the body cannot make on its own. These acids must be obtained through supplements or food.

Two essential elements are omega-3 and omega-6. Omega-6 tends to increase inflammation, while omega-3 helps reduce it. It should be noted that what I wrote earlier is a simplified version of the whole mechanism, and there is much more. Several substances play a more profound role in the entire infrastructure that allows the body to control its incendiary device. Some of the most important are histamine: white blood cells near an injury tend to release a histamine substance. They increase the permeability of blood vessels around the wound, which signals to fight cells and other materials to regulate the immune response and detect injury.

Histamine also causes redness and swelling around the affected area, creating a runny nose, rash, and itchy eyes. Cytokines: These are proteins that are activated by pro-inflammatory eicosanoids to signal the fighting cells to build up at the injury site. They are responsible for diverting energy from the body to catalyze the healing process. The release of these substances tends to cause fatigue and decrease appetite. C-reactive protein: Cytokines and other pro-inflammatory eicosanoids are intimately involved in the activation of a material known as C-reactive protein. This particular organic compound produced by the liver responds to the messages of white blood cells. C-reactive proteins tend to bind to the injury site and act as a kind of monitoring unit that helps identify invading bodies. Leukocytes: Several types of leukocytes (also called white

blood cells) are essential to the process of neutralizing invasive substances. Neutrophils, for example, are small, agile and can first arrive at the crime scene to ingest little germs.
However, large substances such as macrophages are necessary to target a large number of microbes. There are a few others, but the essence remains the same. When your body begins to experience an uncontrolled inflammation attack, the action of these and other similar substances tends to go haywire, which leads to extremely uncomfortable situations. Harmful side effects of inflammation Uncontrolled inflammation produces diseases called autoimmune diseases. Although there are a large number of them, some of the most important is type 1 diabetes: type 1 diabetes can cause the immune system to attack and destroy the disrupting insulin-producing cells in the pancreas regulating sugar levels. in your body. Rheumatoid arthritis: RA causes the immune system to attack certain joints that can cause discomfort and pain. Psoriatic arthritis causes the skin cells to multiply rapidly, causing red, scaly patches on the skin called plaques. Multiple sclerosis: MS tends to damage the protective layer that surrounds nerve cells (known as myelin sheath) and affects the transmission of neural messages between the brain and the body. This leads to weakness, balance problems, and other symptoms. Inflammatory bowel syndromes: this disease irritates the intestinal mucosa. Graves' disease: This disease attacks and overproduces the thyroid gland in the neck, which results in an imbalance. Cancer: cancerous tumors tend to secrete substances that attract cytokines and free radicals that cause inflammation, which can lead to tumor growth. which produces red, scaly patches on the skin called plaques.

If you already have inflammation, this could be the word of the situation. Alzheimer's: the brain has no pain receptors, but that doesn't mean it won't be able to feel the inflammation. Researchers recently discovered that people with high levels of omega-6 fatty acids tend to be more likely to develop Alzheimer's disease. Different Symptoms of Inflammation Although there are different types of illnesses caused by inflammation, the first symptoms are similar. These include Fatigue, Muscle pain, mild fever, redness, and swelling Numbness of the feet and hands Hair loss Rash. They are often accompanied by specific symptoms of any disease the patient may be suffering from.

About the anti-inflammatory diet In general, an anti-inflammatory diet consists of a diet consisting of foods designed to reduce the uncontrolled inflammatory response in the body. The anti-inflammatory diet is rich in foods rich in antioxidants, which are reactive molecules in the menu to help reduce free radicals, causing cellular damage to the body. Many popular diets already follow the anti-inflammatory principle, such as the Mediterranean diet, which consists of fish, good fats, and whole grains.

Chapter 9. Functional Foods for the Anti-Inflammatory Diet

Despite popular belief, following an anti-inflammatory diet is not a challenge. The following foods will support a healthy anti-inflammatory lifestyle: dark green leafy vegetables such as kale and spinach, blueberries, cherries, blackberries, dark red grapes, cauliflower and broccoli, green tea, lentils and red wine (with moderation), avocado and coconut, olives, extra virgin olive oil, nuts, almonds, pistachios, pine nuts, cold-water fish; spices and herbs with salmon and sardines; cinnamon, turmeric, dark chocolate, watermelon, onion, whole grains; brown rice, bulgur, quinoa eggs, tomatoes.

These are just the basics; there is much more to consider.

Harmful foods for anti-inflammatory diet foods to avoid if you want to keep your inflammation under control. Sweet food; soft drinks, baked candies, candies, delicious coffee Vegetable oil products; mayonnaise, barbecue sauce, potato chips, crackers Fried foods; French fries, fish sticks, fried chicken, onion rings Refined flour products; pizza, pasta, flour tortillas, bagels, crackers Dairy products; milk, yogurt, butter, soft cheeses Artificial sweeteners; designates products without added sugars, such as Coca-Cola Light, artificial additives; including breakfast cereals, ice cream, candy, saturated fat; burgers, fries, pizza, and candy Conventional grain-fed meats; beef, pork, chicken Processed meats; bacon, sausage, jerky, gluten sausage from store-bought products; bread, white flour Excess alcohol Trans edible fats; margarine, baked goods like cookies,

Frequently asked Questions

1. Should I detoxify before anti-inflammatory? When you detoxify your body, you are permanently removing harmful toxins that have accumulated in your body. Completing a rehab before you start your anti-inflammatory is a great way to ensure the effectiveness of your new lifestyle.

2. Should I see a doctor for my inflammation? An anti-inflammatory lifestyle is mostly plant-based and requires an individual to skip certain products like dairy and red meat. If you are already on a similar diet, such as a vegan diet, you will have less trouble changing your eating habits. However, if you are taking this step for the first time and trying to change your lifestyle completely, it is recommended that you see a doctor make sure you are in an excellent place to change your eating habits. Alternatively, if you already have an autoimmune disease, it is even more advisable to consult your doctor to create a meal plan based on your needs.

3. Should I exercise more? Having a healthy and fit body certainly helps reduce the risk of problems when you start this new lifestyle. If you are obese, you may face specific inflammatory reactions, so it is best to start with a minimal level of exercise in your daily routine before moving on to a more intense workout.

Chapter 10. Tips for moving to an anti-inflammatory lifestyle

You will need the inspiration to continue when you switch to the anti-inflammatory diet when the tough times come! When you want that ice cream or that bag of crispy fries, but you know you're focusing on health, the tips in this chapter will help you maintain your new healthy lifestyle and beat those cravings.

The first tip to keep in mind is to have an anti-inflammatory vision chart with a graphical representation of your goals for following the anti-inflammatory diet. You can use magazines, newspapers or coupons, or a simple hand-drawn explanation to keep your goals in front of you. At a time of weakness, a glance at your dashboard can be the trick to help you keep going. You can also use social media to identify your favorite anti-inflammatory practitioners and blogs you can refer to for inspiration.

You will also want to consider keeping a food journal. It's a great way to track your progress and celebrate your wins. You can get an old notebook or journal and keep track of what you ate during the day, take notes if you had cravings, and did you give in, or how did you manage it? A food diary will help you observe your eating patterns and what works for you and what doesn't help you maintain the anti-inflammatory lifestyle as effectively as possible.

Set a personal goal to share your trip with someone else. Sharing your journey with others can add more meaning and help others see the benefits of living an anti-inflammatory lifestyle.

Remember to take small steps during your transition. He didn't have chronic inflammation overnight, so you shouldn't expect him to heal overnight. Don't expect to lose 50 pounds in a week. Keep your goals realistic and celebrate your little successes. Remember, this is not a diet; it is a way of life. As long as you stay true to your lifestyle, the results should happen. Remember to keep going, don't stop and let the diet do the work for you.

Do you think about why you eat or eat snacks? This can help you stop eating things that are not right for you.

If you make a mistake, don't be discouraged. Tomorrow is another day. Treat it like that, and go back to your anti-inflammatory horse and put it on. Organize a dinner! This will help others to see what you are doing and will help you on your journey.

Learn the anti-inflammatory equivalent of your favorite recipes from your desserts to your favorite pasta. Also, look for healthy substitutes for what you like.

One serving equals one cup of raw food or half a cup when cooked. A good rule of thumb is to try to eat nine servings of fruits and vegetables each day.

Try at least one recipe or new spice per week. This will help keep your trip fresh and fun. Also, never stop learning. Keep researching and learning about the anti-inflammatory diet so you can continue to get great results.

If you enjoy snacking, try to eat at least two snacks a day. You can also take anti-inflammatory supplements like fish oil or curcumin at this time.

Be prepared! Try to pre-cook your meals so that when you are hungry, you do not slip because you already have food ready. You can also keep small snacks in the places you always visit for easy access to meals.

If you don't like something or a tip doesn't suit you, don't feel guilty for not doing it. An anti-inflammatory diet is one that you can modify and adjust as desired.
Make it a habit to read the ingredient lists. This can help you spot the inflammatory ingredients you didn't know where they were. You can also check your sauces and condiments to see if they cause inflammation or not.
Drink water! Drinking lots of water helps you stay hydrated and can be extremely helpful.
Finally, do you eat as many vegetables and healthy anti-inflammatory foods as possible? When was the last time you heard someone say they got sick from eating so many plants?

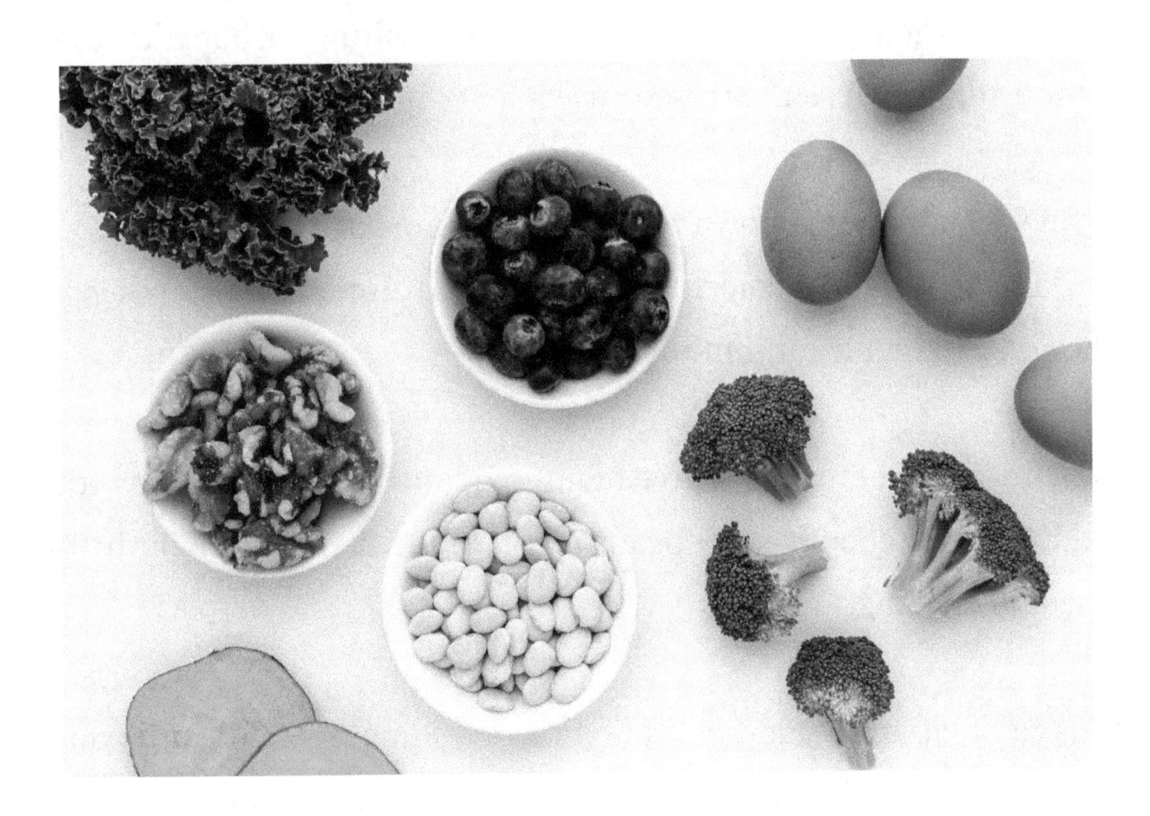

Chapter 11: Foods allowed/avoided

Your diet can significantly affect your immune system. The microbiome (bacteria and microorganisms) in your digestive tract helps regulate your body's natural defense system. Whatever you choose to eat will cause or reduce inflammation.

Choosing to follow a diet with balanced fatty acids will help soothe chronic low-grade inflammation and help you feel better. An essential anti-inflammatory diet focuses on eliminating sugary and processed foods and adding enormous amounts of fresh produce, healthy fats, unprocessed whole grains, spices, and herbs. Limiting carbohydrates is also important because they also cause a lot of inflammation.

Colorful vegetables are known to be a good source of antioxidants. By adding a wide variety of colorful vegetables and eliminating starches, this will help strengthen your immune system.

Legumes are another great source of antioxidants and protein. To reduce the additives, try choosing dry beans and soaking them overnight before rinsing and cooking.

Cereals can help reduce inflammation by providing fiber and antioxidants if you choose the right ones. Many people are sensitive to gluten, even those without celiac disease; This can cause digestive and systemic inflammation. Be sure to choose gluten-free unprocessed grains, such as whole oats, quinoa, barley, and brown rice.

Extra virgin olive oil is high healthy fat and should be your choice when cooking or dressing a salad. Extensive olive oil provides monounsaturated fats, which can be useful for the heart, as well as antioxidants and a compound called oleocanthal, which is known to reduce inflammation. While many foods should be included in your diet to help reduce chronic inflammation, there are also certain foods to avoid to reduce swelling.

Processed foods and sugars are two of the main culprits of inflammation in the Western diet. Processed foods are highly refined, causing them to lose much of their natural fiber and nutrients. They also tend to be high in omega 6, trans fat, and saturated fat, which increases inflammation.

Sugar is one of the worst offenders when it comes to increased inflammation. Not only is it hidden in many foods, but studies have shown it to be very addictive. Thus, you should expect to go through a withdrawal phase when you eliminate it from your diet. This can often cause headaches, cravings, and slowness. Give yourself some time to allow your body to work. Sugar, even natural sugars like honey and agave, causes the body to release cytokines, triggering an immune response that causes inflammation. You don't have to eliminate natural sugars from your diet, but you should only eat them a few times a week, not over one meal a day.

Most fried foods, especially fried foods, should also be avoided.

They are usually cooked in processed oils or lard and coated with refined flour that promotes inflammation.

It would help if you were careful with the foods known as nightshades. Night hats can be anti-inflammatory, but some people are sensitive to them, if it seems like you have more swelling after consuming a night hat, you may want to start making substitutions in your recipes.

Below are many foods that you should increase in your diet, as well as those that you should limit or avoid. This list is not exhaustive, so be sure to stick to the points above.

Food to taste	Foods to avoid
Kale thong	Night shadows like
Beans	Banana peppers
Spinach water	Peppers
chestnut	Thai peppers
Pet	Tomatoes
Arugula fennel	Tomatoes
Lettuce broccoli	Peppers
Carrot peppers	Sweet pepper
Cabbage rhubarb	Habanero
Artichoke shallots	Eggplant
Asparagus mushrooms	Jalapeno
Garlic beetroot	Potatoes (sweet potatoes are good)
Brussels sprouts Onion	
Leeks with zucchini	Artichoke
Pumpkin radish	All canned and frozen vegetables should be avoided.

Watercress thistle BeetrootBok Choy Cucumber celery Turnips **<u>Fruits</u>** Cranberries with apples Watermelon pomegranate Apricot melon Banana plum Pineapple Strawberries Blackberries Cherries Starfruit Pear Papaya dates Orange figs Nectarine grapes Guava Mango Lemon honey Clementine kiwi	**<u>Fruits</u>** All canned and frozen fruit should be avoided.

protein	**protein**
Tempeh soybeans	Dairy
Edamame soy milk	Frozen or processed food
Organic tofu eggs	Non-organic eggs
Protein	**Protein**
Tuna sole	Hormone red meat
Clam shrimp	Processed meats like cold cuts, sausages, bacon and sausages.
Striped rainbow trout	
Sardines snapper	
Halibut Crab	
Herring salmon	
Lobster oysters	
Skinless organic chicken eggs	
Grain	**Grain**
Black barley rice	White rice
Wild rice quinoa	Wheat flour
Oats with brown rice	Corn
Buckwheat millet	
Bulgar Farro	
Corn	

Starchand vegetables	**Starchand vegetables**White potatoes can cause inflammation in people who are sensitive to shadows.
Acorn yam Jicama Butternut To crush Golden potato parsnip Artichokes Red potatoes Pumpkin sweet potatoes Purple potatoes White potatoes	
Fats and oils	**Fats and oils**
Almond avocado Oil Cashew with almond butter Cashew butter with almond oil	Safflower vegetable oil Soybean oil Grapeseed oil Peanut Butter Mayonnaise Corn oil

Hazelnuts in olive oil Chia nuts Sesame seed in walnut oil Oil Hemp seeds Flax seeds Avocado from brazil Pumpkin seed nuts Macadamia nuts Olives Sunflower seed butter	
Herbs and spices Turmeric garlic Cinnamon with ginger Thyme basil Black pepper sage Parsley with coriander Cayenne pepper oregano Mint Dill Cumin clove	Cayenne and chili peppers can cause inflammation in people who are sensitive to shadows.
Beverage's Water Green, black, white, herbal and oolong tea	**Beverage's** All other drinks should be avoided.

White potato: sweet potato, parsnip or turnips. Tomatoes: beets, squash or squash. Peppers: carrots, celery, cucumbers or radishes. Chili pepper and Cayenne Turmeric, black pepper, cloves, ginger or garlic powder. Eggplant - Portobello Mushrooms, Zucchini or Okra.	

Chapter 12

THE 7-DAY ANTI-INFLAMMATORY FOOD PLAN

IN SUMMARY:

• Your food choices are essential to your health and can help reduce inflammation and, therefore, the symptoms it causes.
• In addition to a healthy diet and proper treatment, reducing inflammation can help prevent illnesses and diseases like obesity and heart disease.
• Always choose whole, natural, and unprocessed foods.
• Eat a diet rich in fiber.
• Choose healthy unsaturated fats instead of saturated fats.
• Use herbs and spices for seasoning rather than salt and sugar.
• Eat a variety of colorful fruits and vegetables.
• Vary your diet to include a combination of vitamins and nutrients needed to stay healthy.
• It is not a "weight loss" diet, but it is sturdy and manageable, and you will feel good, and you will likely lose extra pounds during the process.
• The diet will help "flush out" unwanted toxins from your body.
• Stay hydrated and try to drink at least eight glasses of water each day.
• Choose green tea, sparkling water, fruit-infused water, such as lemon or lime water, and very diluted juices, such as pomegranate or cherry juice.
• Drink coffee in moderation and avoid alcohol and soft drinks.

• Choose supplements like a multivitamin. If you don't eat a lot of oily fish, you should also take a fish oil supplement.

WAY OF LIFE:

Exercise is essential and keeps you fit and healthy. However, it is essential not to stress your body too much, as this can cause inflammation. Walking, light jogging, and exercise routines like yoga and pilates are less strenuous but are also rewarding options. Consult your doctor for more information on this subject.

Avoid smoking and drinking too much alcohol. These things may seem rewarding and fun at the moment, but the effects they have on your body and your overall health are not worth it.

7 DAY MEAL PLAN

This meal plan is simple to follow, and the dishes are not too difficult to prepare.

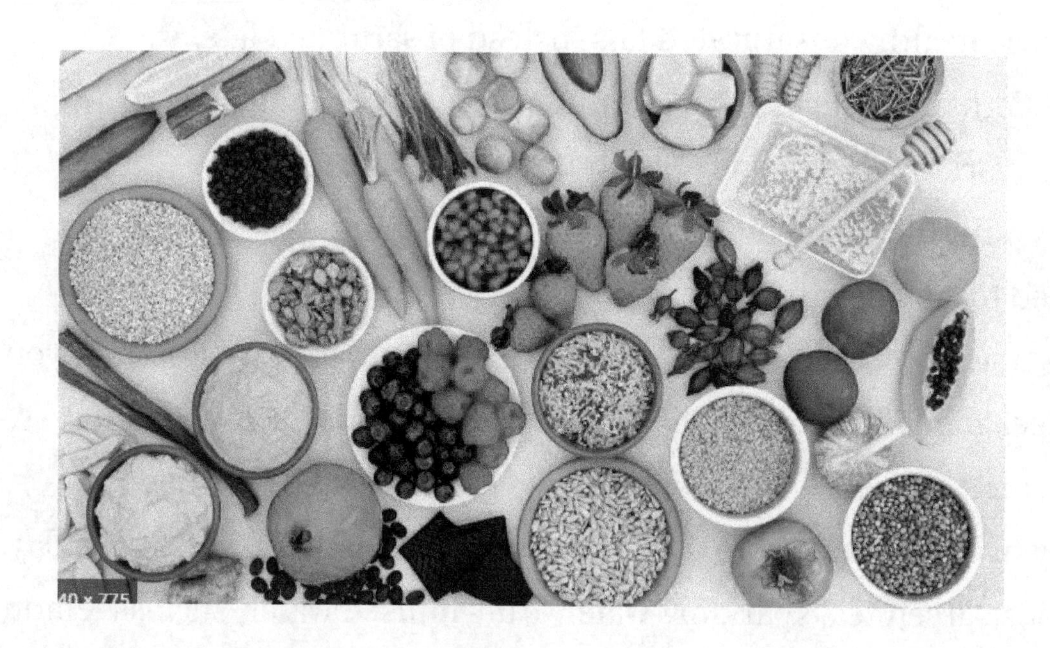

Monday

Drink before breakfast: a glass of lemon water BREAKFAST: coconut breakfast.

LUNCH: Jar of noodles with shrimp and zucchini.

DINNER: Tilapia with nut crust and kale

Tuesday

Drink before breakfast: a glass of lemon water

BREAKFAST: Zucchini and sweet potato frittata

LUNCH: Ginger and spicy carrot soup

DINNER: Baked Garlic Halibut

Wednesday

Meal before breakfast: a glass of lemon water

BREAKFAST: Delicious gluten-free pancakes

LUNCH: tasty Thai broth

DINNER: Vegetable Lasagna

Thursday

Drink before breakfast: a glass of lemon water

BREAKFAST: Blueberry Brain Booster

LUNCH: Burrito Bowl

DINNER: sun-dried tomato paste and nuts

Friday

Drink before breakfast: a glass of lemon or lime water

BREAKFAST: Perfect Punch Fruit Pancakes

LUNCH: Shitake Pumpkin Soup

DINNER: Italian spaghetti with zucchini and chicken

Saturday

Before breakfast: a glass of lemon water.

BREAKFAST: Blueberry and spinach smoothie

LUNCH: Vegetarian tagine

DINNER: Salmon pan on baby arugula

Sunday

Before breakfast: a glass of lemon water

BREAKFAST: avocado boats

LUNCH: Herring salad with celery

DINNER: Spanish shrimp

Snacks

Do not hesitate to choose between 1 and 2 snacks per day between meals. See the Sides and Snacks chapter for ideas.

Chapter 13:Recipes

BREAKFAST:

Sweet Potato Salad

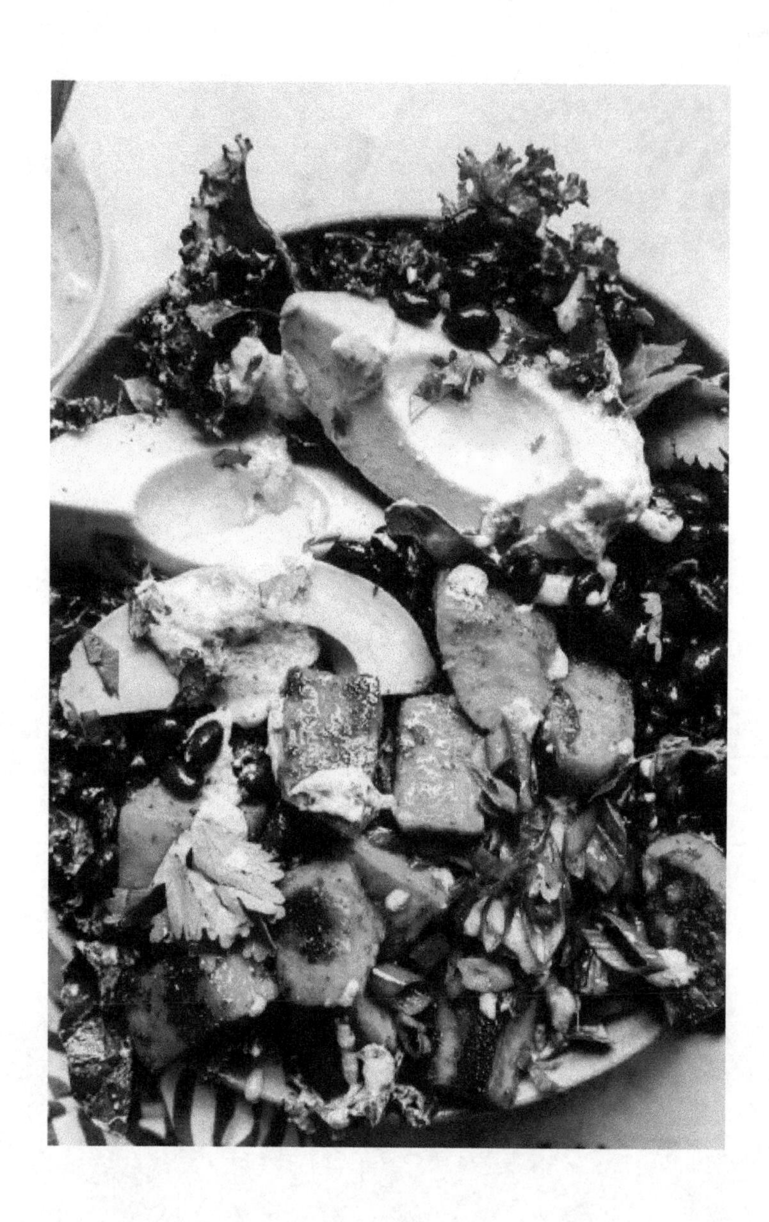

Ingredient

- Baked and cubed sweet potato (1)
- Peeled banana (1)
- Raspberries (.25 c.)
- Raspberries (.25 c.)
- Blueberries (.25 c.)
- Protein powder (1 scoop)

Preparation steps

1. Put a potato in a bowl and mash it with a fork.
2. Add in the protein powder and the banana and mix it all together well.
3. Add in the berries, mix this around, and leave in the fridge a bit before serving.
4. Enjoy

Turkey Hash

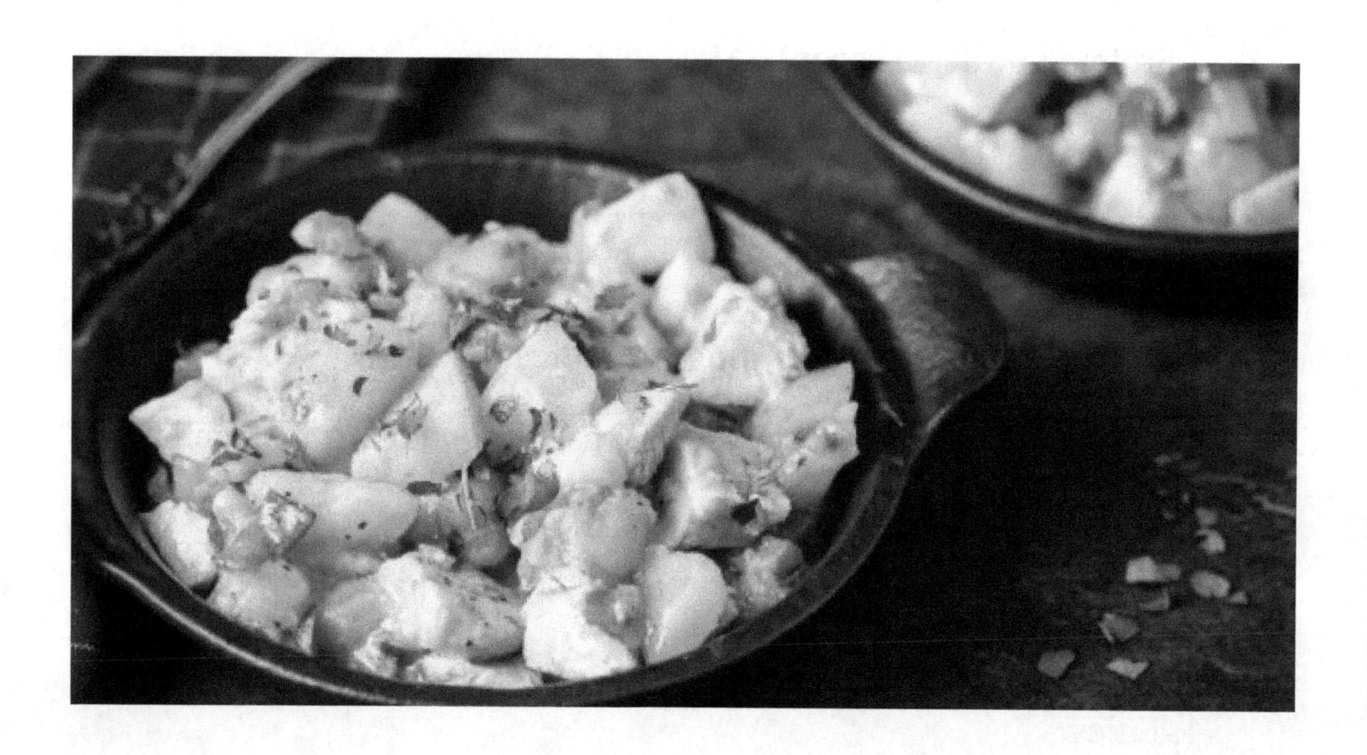

Ingredient

- Ground cinnamon (.5 tsp.)
- Melted coconut oil (1 Tbsp.)
- Dried thyme (.5 tsp.)
- Ground turkey (1 lb.)

For the hash:

- Dried thyme (.5 tsp.)
- Turmeric powder (.5 tsp.)
- Garlic powder (.5 tsp.)
- Ground cinnamon (1 tsp.)
- Ground ginger (1 tsp.)
- Baby spinach (2 c.)
- Cubed apple (1)
- Cubed butternut squash (2 c.)
- Shredded carrots (.5 c.)
- Chopped zucchini (1)
- Melted coconut oil (1 Tbsp.)

Chopped yellow onion (1)

Preparation steps

1. To start this recipe, heat up a pan with some of the coconut. When it is ready, add in the ground turkey with some thyme and cinnamon. Cook to heat up and then move to a bowl.
2. When the turkey is done, heat up some more coconut oil before adding in the onion. Cook for a few minutes before adding in the garlic powder, turmeric, thyme, cinnamon, ginger, apple, squash, carrots, and zucchini.
3. Cook these ingredients around for a bit.
4. After four minutes, add the turkey back into the pan along with the baby spinach. Mix these together to heat up and then serve.
5. Enjoy

Cinnamon Pudding

Ingredient

- Brown rice, uncooked (1 c.)
- Ground cinnamon (1 tsp.)
- Vanilla (1 tsp.)
- Salt
- Maple syrup (.25 c.)
- Coconut or almond milk, unsweetened (3 c.)

How to make

1. To start this recipe, bring out your slow cooker and get it all set up.
2. Add in the salt, maple syrup, milk, and brown rice and mix these ingredients together well.
3. Cover the slow cooker and cook this on a high setting until the rice becomes tender. It will take about three hours.
4. Before serving, stir in the cinnamon and the vanilla and enjoy.

Chia and Strawberry Oats

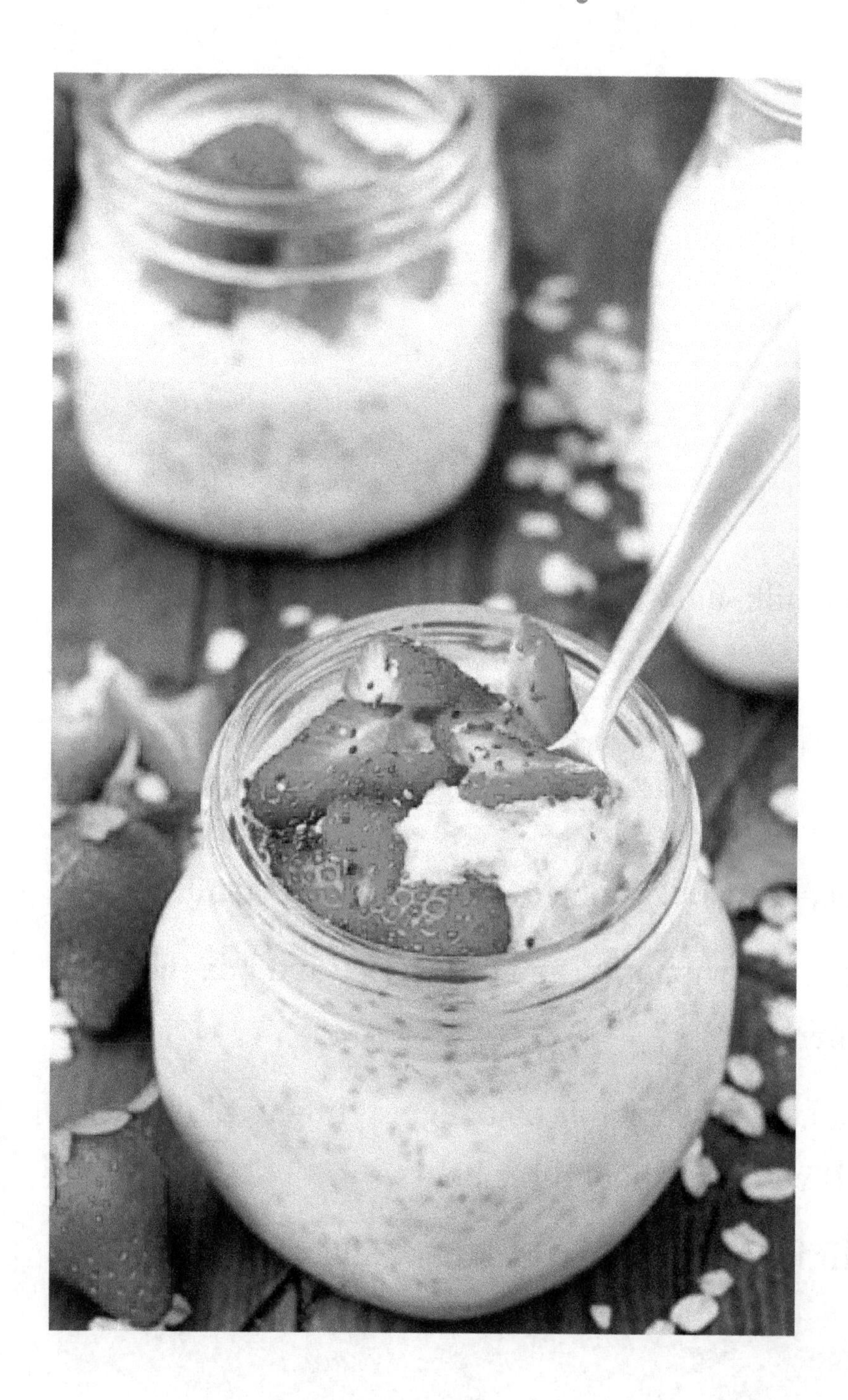

Ingredient

- Toasted oats (.5 c.)
- Vanilla (.5 tsp.)
- Maple syrup (.25 c.)
- Chia seeds (.33 c.)
- Almond milk (2 c.)
- Sliced and peeled kiwi (1)
- Sliced strawberries

How to make

1. Take out a Mason jar of your choice and then add in the vanilla, maple syrup, and chia seeds.
2. Place the lid on top and shake it around well.
3. Set this aside to thicken a bit before. You will need to give it a minimum of 15 minutes to do this, but many times having it in the fridge overnight is the best.
4. When you are ready to serve, take out two serving dishes and divide up the pudding between them.
5. Top the pudding with the toasted oats, kiwi, and strawberries before you serve.
6. Enjoy

Buckwheat Granola

Ingredient

- Vanilla (1 tp.)
- Maple syrup (.25 c.)
- Olive oil (.33 c.)
- Chopped pecans (.5 c.)
- Buckwheat granola (3 c.)
- Salt (.25 tsp.)

Preparation steps

1. Turn on the oven and give it some time to heat up to 350 degrees.
2. While the oven heats up, take out a bowl and combine together the salt, vanilla, syrup, oil, pecans, and buckwheat.
3. Mix these ingredients together well to make sure the buckwheat gets covered with the syrup and oil well.
4. Spread this out over a rimmed baking sheet and put it into the oven to cook for a bit.

5. After 5 minutes, take the sheet out of the oven and stir the oats around. Place back in the oven.
6. After another five minutes, take the sheet out and give it some time to cool down before you serve.
7. Enjoy

Easy Frittata

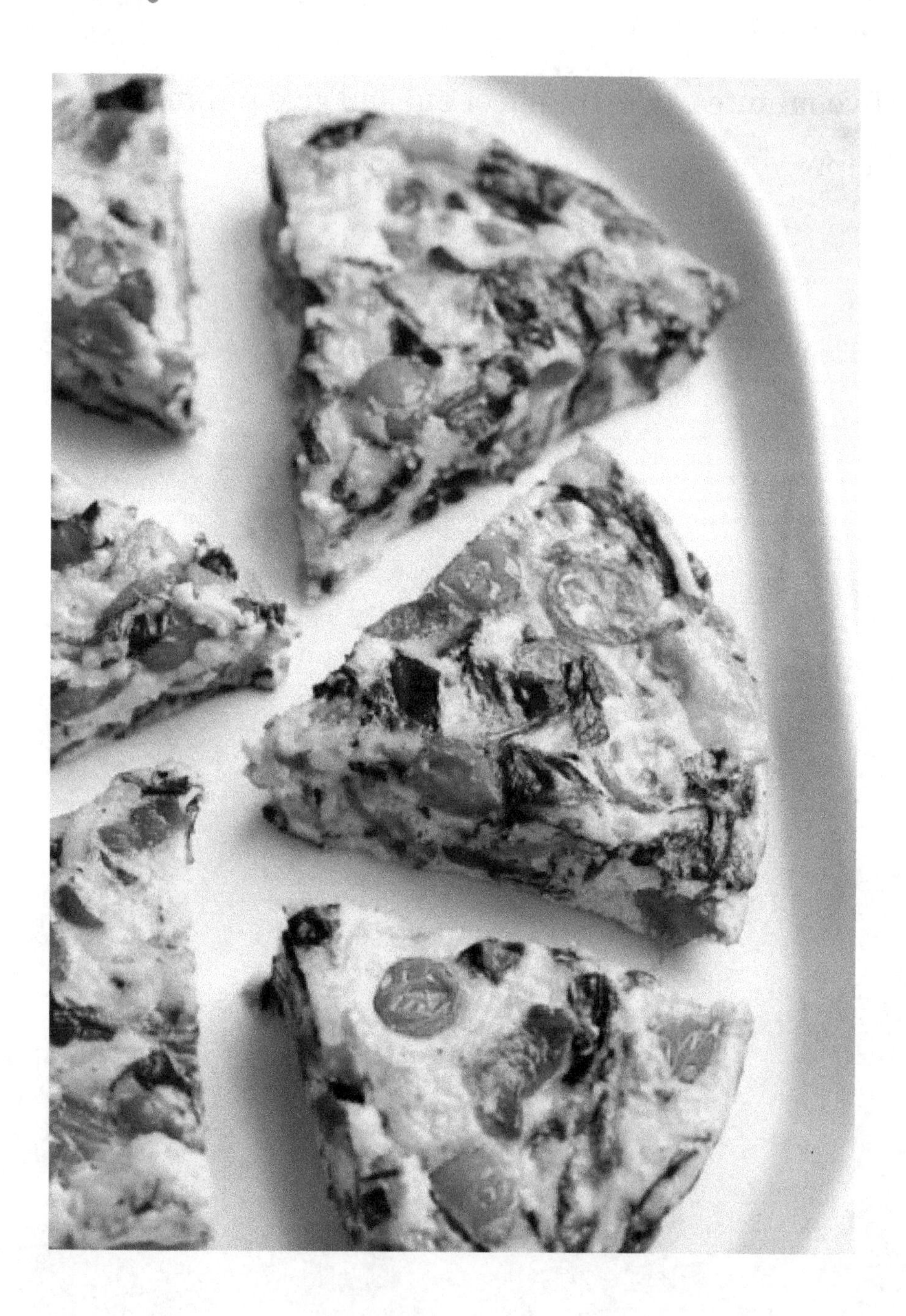

Ingredient

- Chopped sage (1 tsp.)
- Ground cumin (.5 tp.)
- Ground turmeric (1 tsp.)
- Salt (1 tsp.)
- Garbanzo bean flour (1.5 c.)
- Sliced scallions (2)
- Sliced zucchini (1)
- Olive oil (2 Tbsp.)
- Water (1.5 c.)

Preparation steps

1. Turn on the oven and allow it some time to heat up to 350 degrees.
2. While the oven is heating up, take out a bowl and whisk together the sage, cumin, turmeric, salt, and garbanzo bean flour.
3. When you are ready, slowly add in the water. You also want to keep stirring during this time to ensure that the batter is not going to become lumpy. Then set it to the side.
4. Bring out your skillet and heat up some oil on the oven. Cook the zucchini for a bit to help it soften.
5. Stir in the scallions to heat up, and then spoon the batter on top of these vegetables.

6. Place this prepared skillet in the oven and let it bake. After 20 minutes, take the frittata out of the oven and let it cool down before you serve.
7. Enjoy

LUNCH:

Salmon Salad

What's inside

- Chopped dill (1 tsp.)
- Pepper (.25 tsp.)
- Salt (1 tsp.)
- Lemon juice (2 Tbsp.)
- Olive oil (.25 c.)
- Sliced avocado (1)
- Salmon fillets (2)
- Sliced and trimmed fennel bulb (1)
- Sliced cucumber (.5)
- Baby spinach (3 c.)

How to make

1. Take out a big bowl or a serving platter and arrange the spinach inside of it.
2. Top this with the avocado, salmon, fennel, and cucumber.
3. In a second bowl, whisk together the dill, pepper, salt, lemon juice, and olive oil. Stir around well.

4. Pour the dressing on top of the salad and then serve well.
5. Enjoy

Roasted Chicken

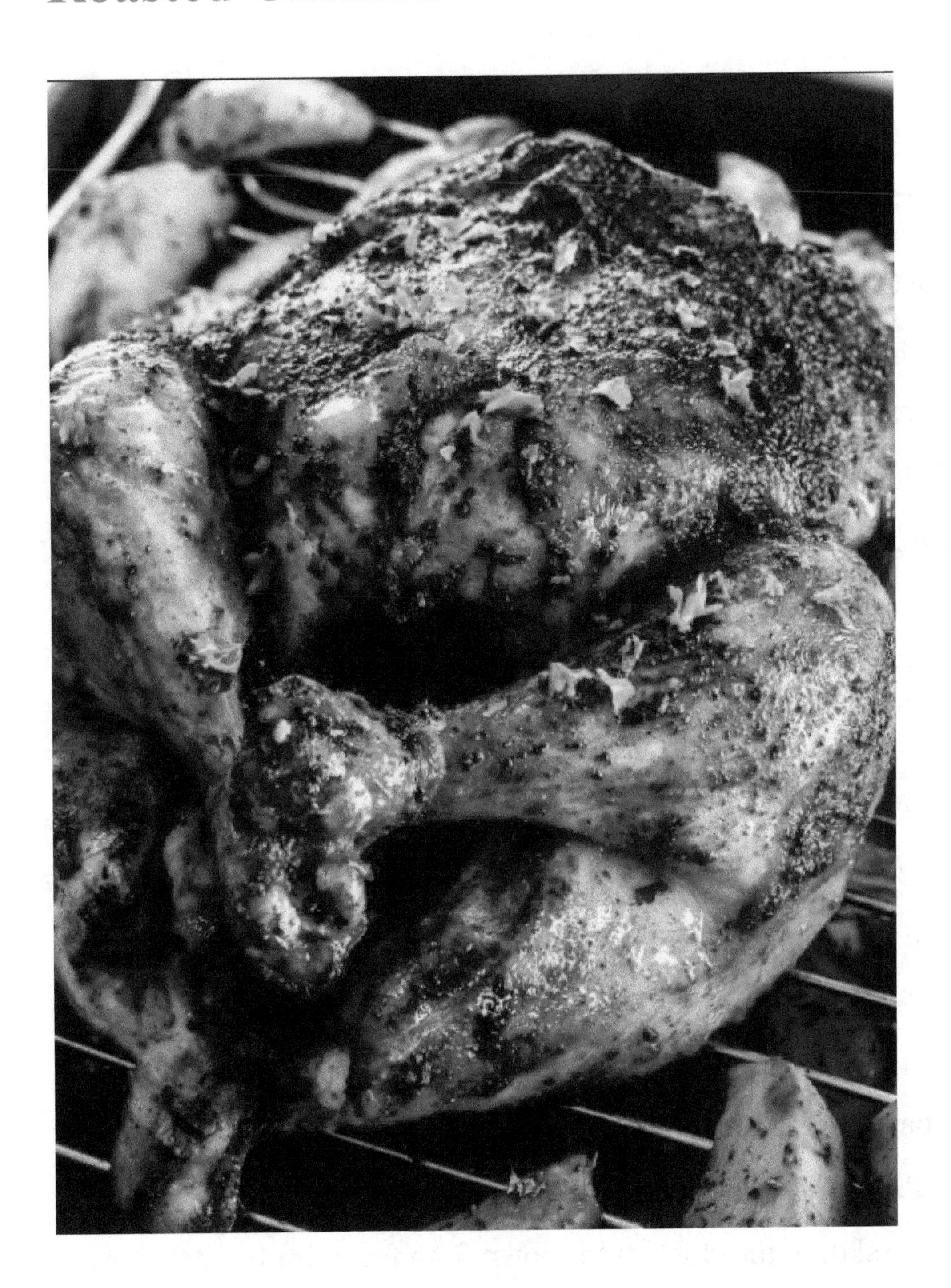

Ingredient

- Pepper
- Salt
- Chicken (4 lb.)
- Olive oil (1 Tbsp.)
- Lemon juice (2 Tbsp.)
- White beans (1 can)
- Dry white wine (.5 c.)
- Chicken broth (.5 c.)
- Sliced garlic cloves (2)
- Sliced onion (1)

Preparation steps

1. Turn on the oven and give it time to heat up to 375 degrees. While the oven is heating up, take out a big Dutch oven and heat up some olive oil inside of it.
2. Use a paper towel to pat the chicken dry before adding on the salt and pepper. Place the chicken into the Dutch oven.
3. Allow the skin of the chicken to brown for a few minutes. After five minutes, turn the chicken over and brown on the other side.
4. Add in the garlic and onion all around the chicken and add in the white wine and broth as well.

5. Place the lid on top of the Dutch oven and then bake for an hour.
6. After this time is up, add in the lemon juice and the white beans. Put the lid back on top and then cook a bit longer.
7. After half an hour, uncover the Dutch oven and give the chicken some time to cool down before serving.
8. Enjoy

Green Smoothie

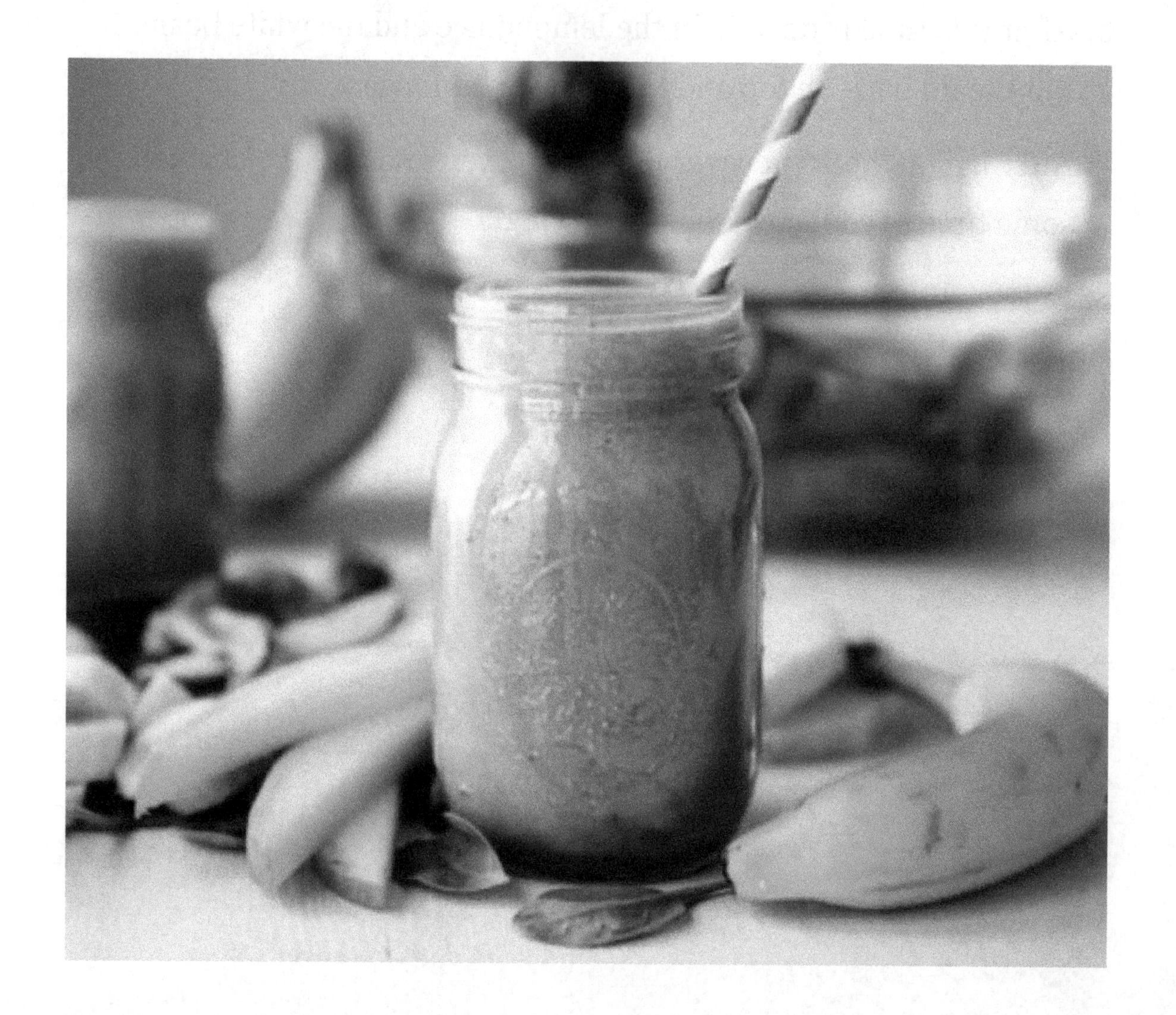

Ingredient

- Ice (.5 c.)
- Almond milk, unsweetened (1 c.)
- Cinnamon (.25 tsp.)
- Maple syrup (1 Tbsp.)
- Green apple (.5)
- Packed baby spinach (1 c.)

How to make

1. Take out your blender and get it all set up.
2. Add all of the ingredients into the blender and turn it on. Blend to make smooth and then serve.
3. Add in some raw pistachios to this if you would like to boost the protein and add a nice buttery flavor to it.
4. Enjoy

Breakfast Salad

Ingredient

- Pepper
- Grated ginger (1 tsp.)
- Minced garlic cloves (1)
- Lemon juice (1 Tbsp.)
- Turmeric powder (1 tsp.)
- Apple cider vinegar (2 Tbsp.)
- Olive oil (.25 c.)
- Cooked and cubed beats (15 oz.)
- blueberries (1.5 c.)
- Kale mixed with dried fruit (27 oz.)

Preparation steps

1. Bring out a salad bowl and mix together the blueberries, beets, dried fruits, and kale.
2. In a second bowl, mix together the pepper, ginger, garlic, lemon juice, turmeric, vinegar, and oil.
3. Enjoy

Whisk the second bowl together well and then pour it on top of the salad before serving and enjoying

Brown Rice Bowl

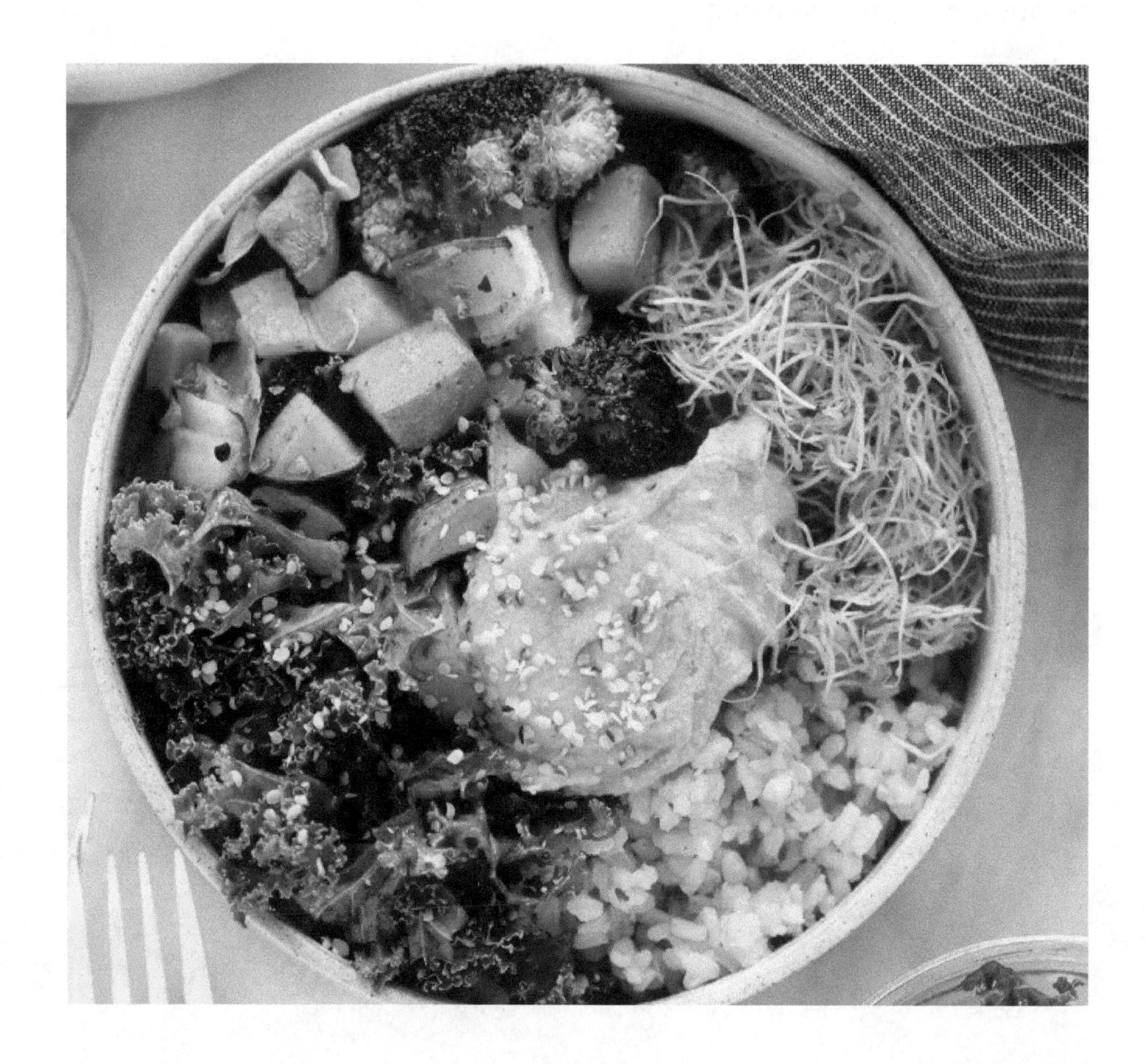

Ingredient

- Sliced carrot (.5)
- Sliced beat (1)
- Sliced cucumber (.5)
- Baby spinach (2 c.)
- Cooked brown rice (4 c.)
- Ginger turmeric dressing (.5 c.)
- Cilantro, chopped (.25 c.)
- Raw cashews (.5 c.)
- Sliced avocado (1)
- Canned lentils (1.)

Sliced red onion (.5)

How to make

1. Take your rice and split it up among four bowls to make the servings.
2. Add the spinach all over the rice along with the avocado, lentils, red onion, carrot, beet, and cucumber.
5. Sprinkle the cilantro and cashews on top before topping it all with some dressing and serving.
6. Enjoy

Mushroom Pasta

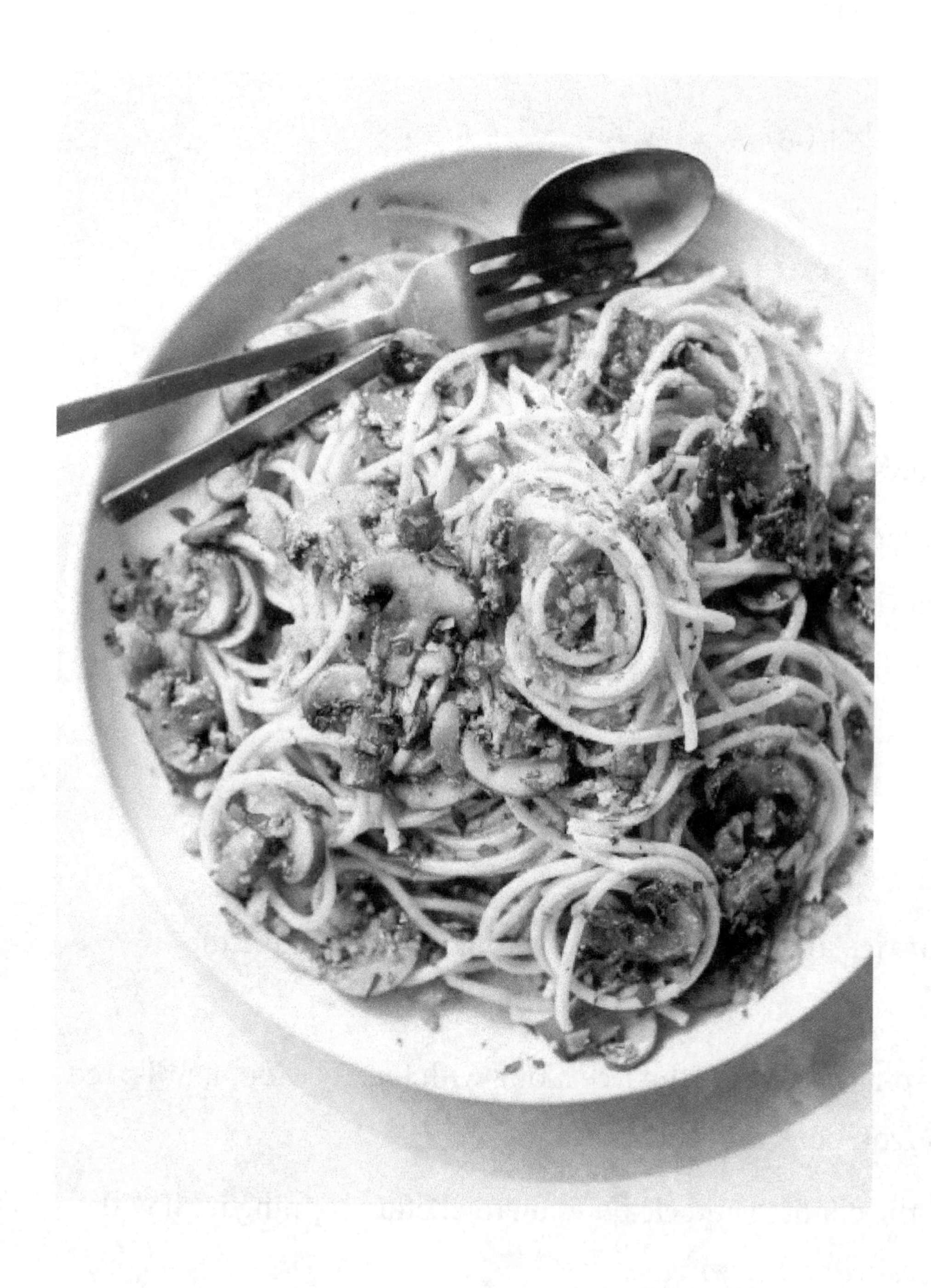

Ingredient

- Dry red wine (.25 c.)
- Ground pepper (.25 tsp.)
- Salt (1 tsp.)
- Cremini mushrooms (2 c.)
- Olive oil (2 Tbsp.)
- Chopped rosemary (1 tsp.)
- Water (4 c.)
- Rigatoni (12 oz.)
- Minced garlic cloves (1)
- Minced shallot (1)

Preparation steps

1. To start this recipe, take out your Dutch oven and heat up some olive oil. Once the oil has some time to heat up, you can add in the red wine, pepper, salt, and mushrooms.
2. Cook this around, stirring occasionally, until the mushrooms have time to cook.
3. After this, add in the garlic, shallot, four cups of water, and the rigatoni. Bring all of these ingredients to a boil.
4. Reduce this to a simmer, cover, and then let the pasta cook to become tender.

5. After another 15 minutes, you can transfer this to a serving bowl and drizzle on the oil and rosemary before serving.
6. Enjoy

Apple and Chicken Salad

Ingredient

- Chopped and toasted walnuts (.5 c.)
- Lemony mustard dressing (.5 c.)
- Canned chickpeas (.5 c.)
- Chopped scallions (3)
- Chopped romaine lettuce heart (1)
- Chopped green apple (1)
- Chopped celery (.5 c.)
- Chicken breasts (2 cooked)

Preparation steps

1. Bring out a bowl and combine together the scallions, romaine, apple, celery, chicken and the chickpeas.
2. Add the dressing to this bowl and then toss it all around to mix.
3. When you are ready to serve, divide up this salad between four bowls and top with the walnuts before serving.
4. Enjoy

Orange Chicken Salad

Ingredient

- Pepper
- Salt
- Toasted cashews (1 c.)
- Coconut cream (.5 c.)
- Avocado mayo (.25 c.)
- Mandarin orange, chopped (1 c.)
- Chopped celery (2)
- Chopped scallions (4)
- Sliced chicken (1 whole)

Preparation steps

1. Bring out a big pot and add in some water. Add the chicken and some salt to this and bring it to a boil.
2. Cook this for a bit. After 25 minutes, take the chicken out of the pot, put it on a cutting board, and get rid of the bones.
3. Shred up the meat and put into a bowl. When the chicken is ready, add in the coconut cream, mayo, pepper, salt, scallions, cashews, orange pieces, and celery.
4. Toss this mixture around to coat and then serve.

5. Enjoy

Chicken and Brown Rice Mix

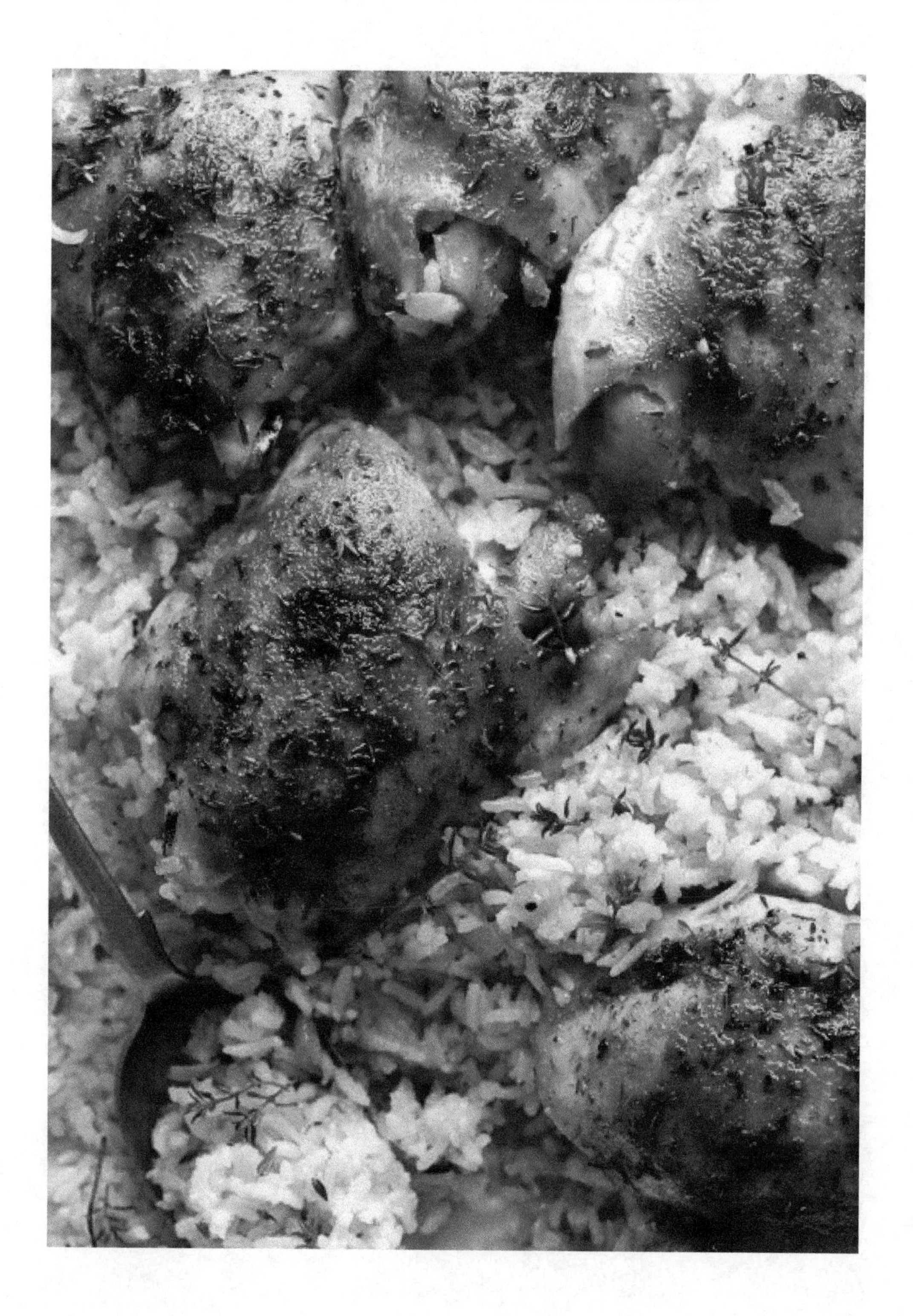

Ingredient

- Chopped scallions (2)
- Egg whites (2)
- Egg (1)
- Sliced chicken breasts (4)
- Coconut aminos (2 Tbsp.) Chicken
- stock (1 c.)
- Coconut sugar (1.5 Tbsp.)
- Cooked brown rice (1.5 c.)

Preparation steps

1. Take out a big pot and add the stock inside. Add to the stove and heat up on a medium low heat.
2. Add in the sugar and the coconut aminos and then stir to bring to a boil. Add in the chicken and toss as well.
3. In a different bowl, mix together the egg whites and the eggs. Whisk these well and then add over the chicken mix.
4. Sprinkle on the scallions over all of this and then cook for a few minutes without stirring.
5. Divide your brown rice into four servings and then add the chicken on the top before serving.
6. Enjoy

Easy Potato and Chicken Mixture

Ingredient

- Canned artichokes (14 oz.)
- Chopped basil (2 Tbsp.)
- Chopped basil (2 Tbsp.)
- Kalamata olives (.25 c.)
- Chopped tomato (2 c.)
- Pepperoncini peppers, chopped (.5 c.)
- Vegetable stock (.75 c.)
- Sliced red onion (1 c.)
- Chicken breast cubed (2 lbs.)
- Cooking spray
- Small red potatoes (12)
- Dried thyme 25 tsp.)
- Pepper
- Salt
- Minced garlic (4 tsp.)

Olive oil (1 Tbsp.)

Preparation steps

1. To start this recipe, turn on the oven and let it have time to heat up to 400 degrees.
2. While the oven is warming up, add the potatoes in a bowl with the pepper, salt, thyme, olive oil, and some garlic. Add to a baking sheet and place into the oven.
3. After 30 minutes, the potatoes are done. Take them out of the oven to cool.
4. Bring out a big pot and grease with the cooking spray. Add in the chicken and then season with some pepper and salt.
5. Cook the chicken for a few minutes on each side and then move to a plate.
6. Heat up that pot again before adding in the onion and cook a bit longer. Add in the chicken and the stock.
7. Now you can add in the potatoes, pepperoncini and olives. Cook for a few minutes before adding in the tomatoes, basil, artichokes, and garlic.
8. When these are all warmed up and ready to go, divide up between your plates and serve.

DINNER:

Balsamic Chicken

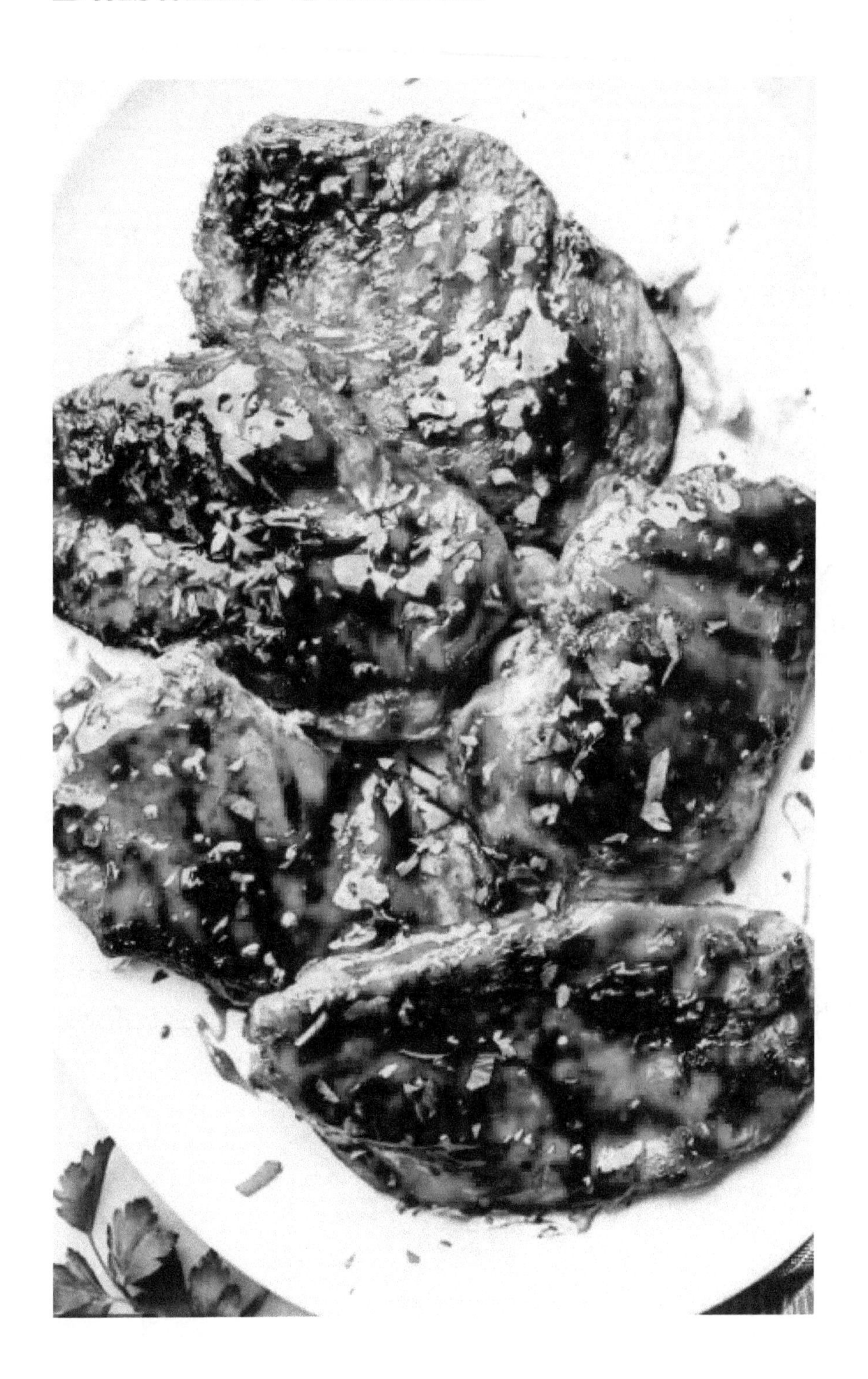

Ingredient

- Chicken breasts (4)
- Salt (1 tsp.)
- Minced shallot (1)
- Honey (2 Tbsp.)
- Balsamic vinegar (.5 c.)

Preparation steps

1. To start this recipe, turn on the oven and let it have time to heat up to 350 degrees.
2. Combine the salt, shallot, honey, and balsamic vinegar inside a baking pan and stir so that the honey is able to dissolve well.
3. Add in the chicken to this mixture and turn it around to coat well. Then add the baking dish to the oven.
4. After 20 minutes, the chicken should be cooked all the way through. Take it out of the oven and let it cool down for a few minutes before slicing and serving.

Turkey Taco Soup

Ingredient

- Salt (1 tsp.)
- Minced garlic cloves (2)
- Sliced zucchini (1)
- Ground turkey (1 lb.)
- Olive oil (1 Tbsp.)
- Chicken broth (4)
- Frozen corn 1 c.)
- Fire roasted tomatoes (1 can)
- Black beans (1 can)
- Pepper
- Cumin

Chipotle pepper (1 tsp.)

Preparation steps

1. Bring out the Dutch oven and heat up some oil on a high heat. When this is nice and warm, add in the ground turkey and let it cook until browned well.
2. At this time, add in the pepper, cumin, chipotle pepper, salt, garlic, and zucchini.

3 After five minutes of those marinating, add in the corn, broth, tomatoes, and black beans to the mix.

4. Bring all of this to a boil and when it gets hot, turn it down to a simmer. Simmer for a few minutes to let the flavors all combine together well.

5. At this time, ladle the soup into bowls and serve, adding on some more toppings if you choose.

6. Enjoy

Feta and Chickpea Casserole

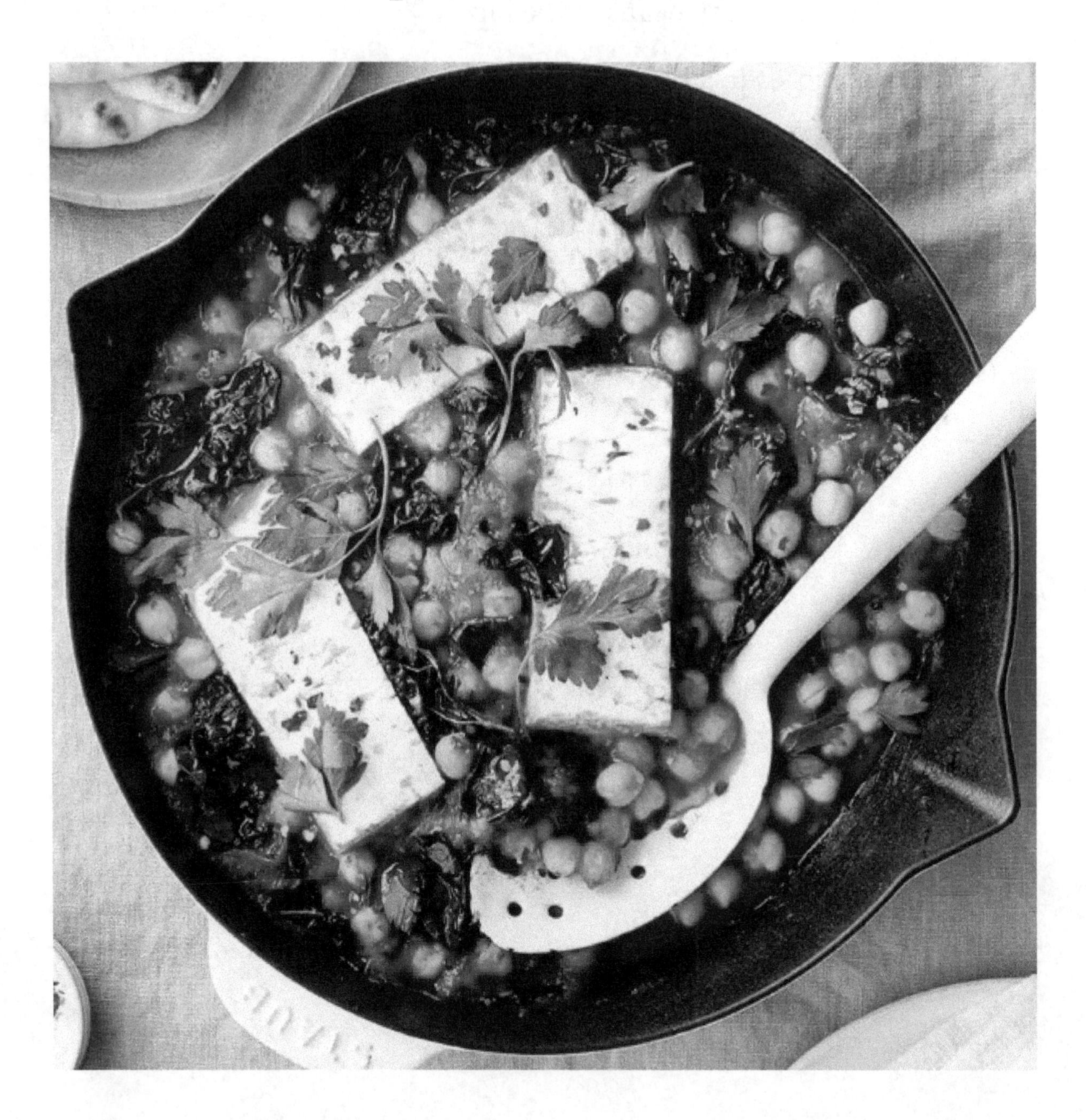

Ingredient

- Chopped garlic cloves (2)
- Chopped zucchini (1)
- Chopped onion (1)
- Olive oil (2 Tbsp.)
- Beaten eggs (4)
- Pepper
- Salt
- Cumin (.5 tsp.)
- Dried oregano (1 tsp.)
- Crumbled feta cheese (.5 c.)
- Chickpeas (1 can)

Preparation steps

1. Turn on the oven and give it some time to heat up. While the oven is warming up, use some olive oil to grease up a baking pan.
2. Now bring out a skillet and heat up a little olive oil on a high heat. When the oil is warm, add in the garlic, zucchini, and onion and let them cook until they start to brown.

3 After five minutes, move the vegetables over to a big bowl along with the chickpeas.

4. Using your potato masher, mash up these vegetables and chickpeas a little bit.
5. When that is done, add in the eggs, pepper, salt, cumin, oregano, and feta and mix them together well.
6. Spoon this mixture into the pan that you have prepared, smooth out the top and add into the oven.
7. After 20 minutes, the dish is done. Take it out of the oven and let it have some time to cool down before serving.
8. Enjoy

Chicken Stir-Fry

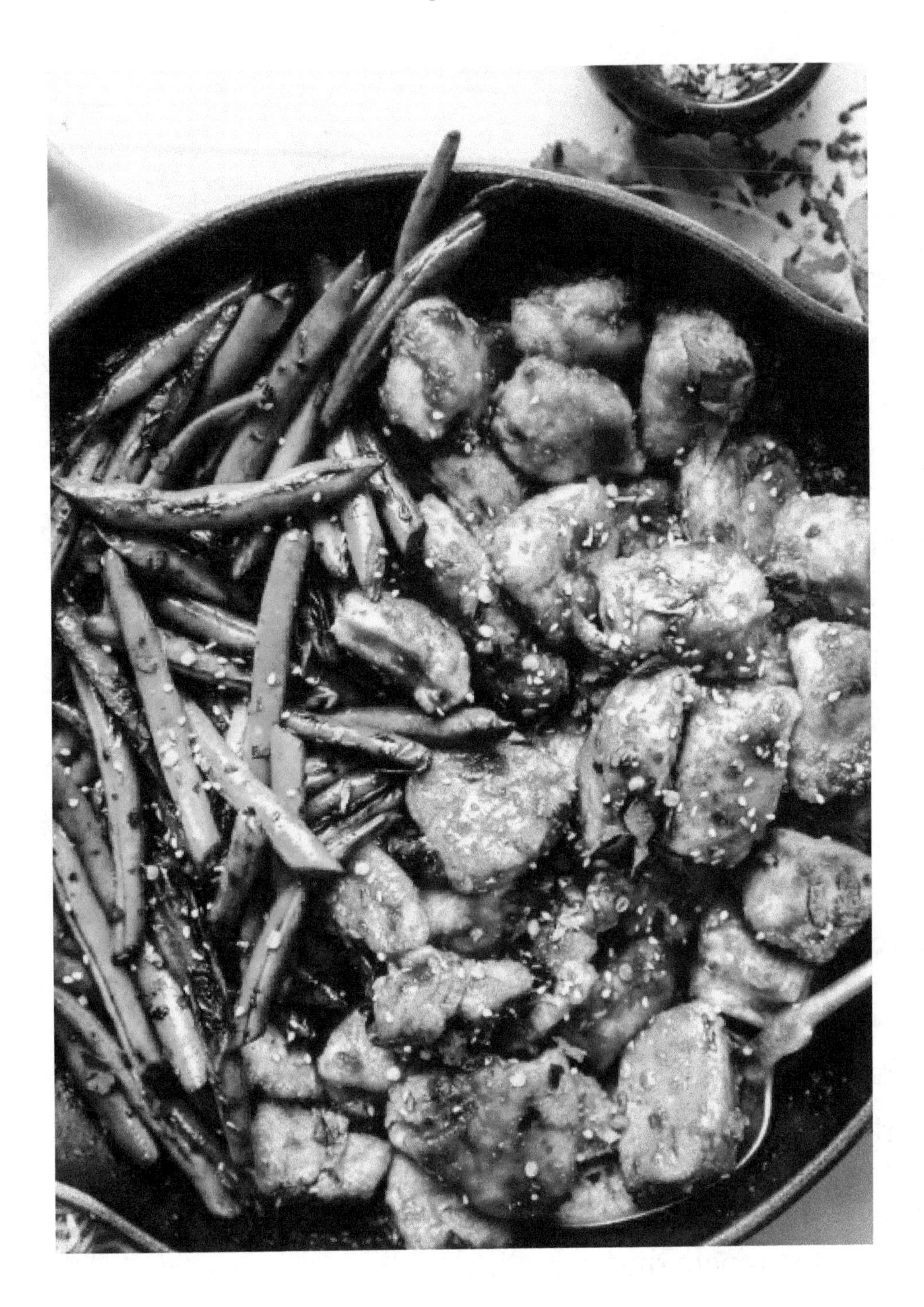

Ingredient

- Chicken thighs (1 lb.)
- Coconut oil (2 Tbsp.)
- Sesame seeds (1 Tbsp.)
- Toasted sesame oil (1 tsp.)
- Chicken broth (.75 c.)
- Red pepper flakes (.25 tsp.)
- Salt (1 tsp.)
- Ginger root, minced (1 tsp.)
- Sliced garlic cloves (2)
- Broccoli florets (2 c.)

How to make;

1. Take out your Dutch oven and heat up the coconut oil on a high eat.
2. Add in the chicken when the oil is hot and cook until it has time to brown. After five minutes, add in the broth, red pepper flakes salt, ginger, garlic, and broccoli.
3. Cover the pot and then lower the heat to a medium. Let the mixture steam for a bit to prepare the broccoli.

4 Remove this from the heat at this time (about five minutes) and add in the sesame seeds and sesame oil. Serve warm.

Garlic Mustard Steak

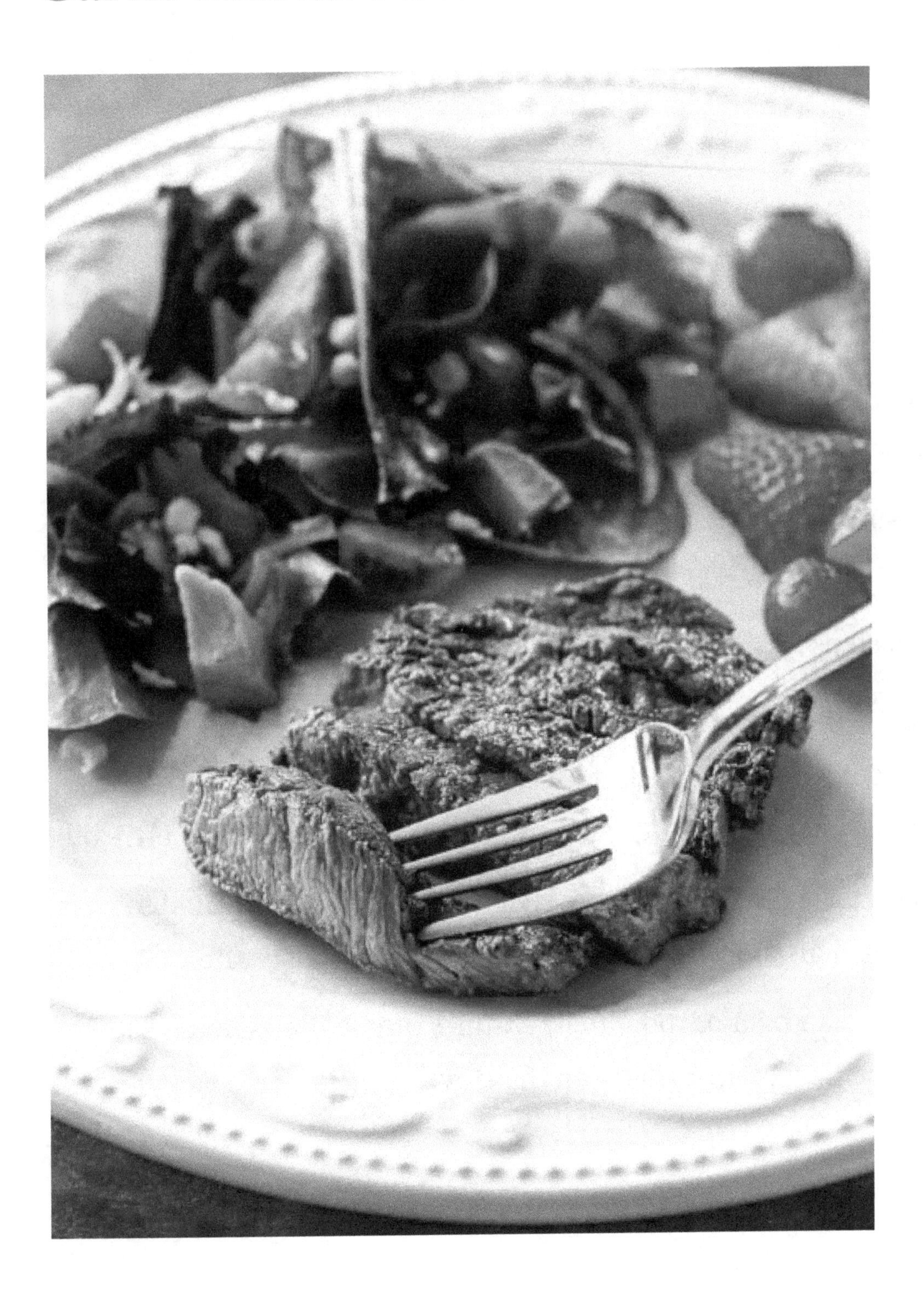

Ingredient

- Chopped rosemary (1 tsp.)
- Minced garlic cloves (2)
- Dijon mustard (2 Tbsp.)
- Balsamic vinegar (.5 c.)
- Olive oil (.5 c.)
- Steaks (4)
- Pepper (.25 tsp.)
- Salt (1 tsp.)

Preparation steps

1. Bring out a baking dish that is shallow and whisk together the pepper, salt, rosemary, garlic, Dijon balsamic vinegar, and olive oil.
2. When that is ready, add in the steaks and turn them around to coat with the marinade. Cover the dish and let these marinate.
3. After half an hour at room temperature, or two hours in the fridge, it is time to heat up a skillet on the stove.

4 Take the steaks out of the marinade and blot them with a paper towel to help get rid of the extra marinade.

5. Cook the steaks, flipping them over once, until they are browned nicely.

6. Allow the teaks five minutes to rest before you serve.

Stuffed Eggplant

Ingredient

- Olive oil (2 Tbsp.)
- Pepper
- Salt
- Ground turmeric (.25 tsp.)
- Sweet paprika (.25 tsp.)
- Lemon juice (1 Tbsp.)
- Chopped oregano (1 Tbsp.)
- Ground turkey (1 lb.)
- Minced garlic cloves (2)

Halved eggplants (6)

Preparation steps

1. To start this recipe, heat up some oil in a pan. When the oil is warm, you can add in the ground turkey and then cook for a bit.
2. After five minutes, add in the turmeric, pepper, salt, paprika, lemon juice, and oregano. Cook for a bit longer.

3. Take this off the heat and give it some time to cool down. Use this mixture to stuff the eggplants and then place them on a prepared baking sheet.
4. Turn on the oven and give it time to heat up to 400 degrees. After it has had time to heat up, then add in the baking sheet.
5. The eggplants are going to be done after half an hour. Divide this between a few plates and then serve.
6. Enjoy

Quinoa and Salmon Salad

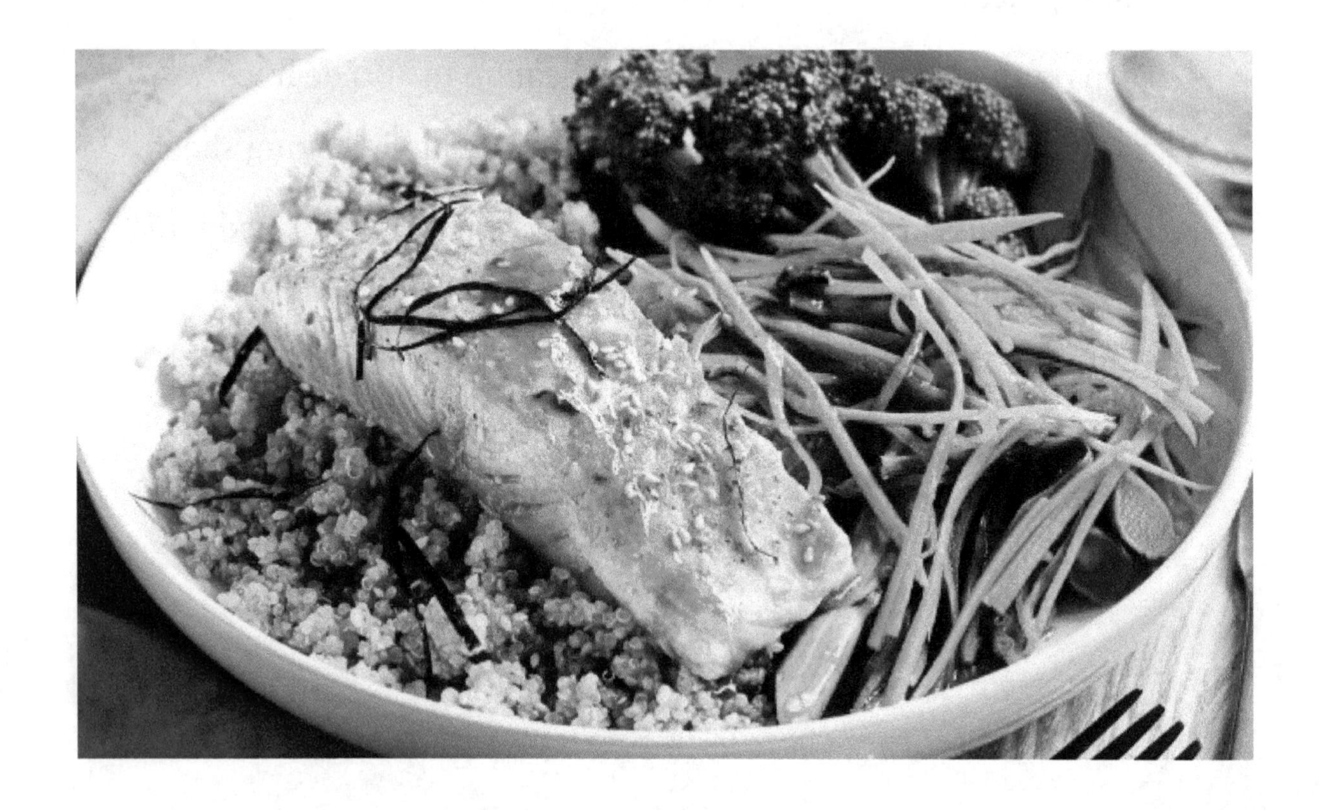

Ingredient

- Salmon fillets (4)
- Hemp seeds (1 Tbsp.)
- Dried currants (.25 c.)
- Canned chickpeas (2 c.)
- Pepper
- Salt
- Olive oil (1 Tbsp.)
- Minced garlic cloves (2)
- Water (2 c.)
- Sliced carrot (1)
- Lemon juice (2 Tbsp>)
- Torn kale (1 bunch)

Rinsed white quinoa (1 c.)

For the sauce

- Coconut cream (.5 c.)
- Lemon juice (1 Tbsp.)
- Tahini paste (.25 c.)
- Water (.5 c.)

Preparation steps

1. Bring out a pot and add in two cups of water along with the quinoa and let this simmer on a medium heat. Cook for 15 minutes and then set aside for a bit to cool down.
2. After that time is up, use a fork to fluff up the quinoa and set to the side.
3. Mix together the quinoa along with the hemp seeds, lemon juice, kale, currants, chickpeas, garlic, and carrot.
4. In a second bowl, combine half a cup of water with the coconut cream, lemon juice, and tahini. Whisk this well and then add it in with the quinoa mix.
5. Toss the mix and set it to the side to marinate for a few minutes.
6. During this time, heat up some olive oil in a pan. When it is hot, add in the salmon, seasoning with some pepper and salt.
7. Cook the salmon for a few minutes on each side. Divide the cooked salmon between a few plates and top with some of the quinoa mixture. Serve this warm and enjoy!